FitMentality

The Ultimate Guide to Stop Binge Eating:

Achieve the Mindset for the

Fit Body You Want

Legal Disclaimer

The publisher as well as the author of this book advise readers to take full and proper responsibility for their safety and physical health and acknowledge their limits as it relates to exercise and nutrition. Prior to practicing the physical activity exercise in this book, ensure that your equipment is suitable and well-maintained. Be advised to refrain from taking any risks beyond your level of fitness experience, training, and aptitude. The dietary and physical activity programs in this book are not intended as a substitute for any physical activity routine or dietary regimen that might have been prescribed by your medical treatment team. As will all physical activity exercises and dietary programs, it is highly recommended that you first seek your medical doctor's approval before beginning a new dietary or exercise regimen.

Contents

Acknowledgements

Thank you Mom. You are my real-life hero. Thank you Dad for your love and support. Thank you brothers for being so wonderful. Thank you Grandma Barbara, Grandpa Chronister, and Grandma Marlene for being so incredible. Thank you to my wonderful Aunts Cherylee and Cindy. Thank you to all of my friends that have been supportive ever since the beginning of my career. Thank you Griselda for your endless support. Thank you to every one of my past, present, and future mentors. Finally, thank you to every single person who has ever reached out to me for help. You have made me a better person and better at helping others.

Introduction

This book is for those who have failed before many times when it comes to recovering from binge eating behaviors. You may be at the point where it feels like this problem is permanent. I have tremendous respect for you for committing yourself to this change. You may be nervous and you may be excited. I do want you to have a positive expectancy. You may not have achieved your goals before, however, this book will take you step by step with achievable steps to guide you to achieve the mindset for the fit body you want.

I am trained in clinical psychology with a specialty in eating disorders including Binge Eating Disorder (BED). It was extremely important for me to write and release this book based on what I know is *not* known widely by the general public. I believe that everyone (not just therapists and psychiatrists and patients at psychiatric hospitals) needs to have access to evidence-based information and tools that can be utilized to eliminate binge eating behaviors.

Before entering the field of psychology, I worked with clients as a certified personal trainer. I cannot tell you how frustrating it is to encounter numerous clients that would sabotage their weight loss goals by overeating. No matter how much physical training you can put a client through it will do absolutely no good if they go home and take in the same or more number of calories they burned earlier that day during a training session. Studies show that working out can give people a false sense of permission to overeat. The truth is, at that time it was painful for me to watch them self-sabotage.

In psychiatric hospitals, I've assessed hundreds of patients struggling with binge eating behaviors. The most memorable assessment that comes to mind was a woman who believed she had lost all hope. She was on disability for mental health and physical health complications as a result of binge eating that had resulted in obesity. She had metabolic issues such as diabetes and she was limited in her mobility. Her EKG was abnormal as the eating had begun to put a strain on her heart. She told me that she loved her family but she didn't care about doing anything for herself and she had lost almost all hope.

She couldn't drive anymore because of her physical state. She said she would be picking up fast food at restaurants all day if she was able to drive. All of the things that brought her joy involved getting out of the house and her depression and physical state would no longer allow her to engage (at least this is what her limiting beliefs allowed her to believe). The consequences became so severe that she decided to call around to inpatient eating disorder psychiatric hospital programs that day. Luckily, her insurance checked out and she made reservations to fly in for treatment for Binge Eating Disorder later that same month.

Not every one of us is obese as a result of overeating and everyone who binge eats does not necessarily fit the diagnosis for Binge Eating Disorder (BED). Binge eating behaviors strike individuals of all ages, shapes, cultures, and sizes. Binge eating can be seen in students, stay-at-home parents, CEOs, adolescents, children, and even athletes (this list is by no means exhaustive). Most of us are not immune to an occasional emotional eating episode and binge eaters lie on a spectrum ranging from occasional binge eaters to extreme binge eaters.

It is well known in the psychology world that many therapists are drawn to one field or another because of personal experience with that disorder such as a family member that struggled with that particular issue. I, myself, went through times in my late adolescence when I lacked meaning and purpose and had strong urges to overeat. In fact, that was one of the reasons I took up personal training in my 20's. I wanted to take back control of my body as I was when I was an athletic child. I wanted to increase my energy levels, increase my confidence, and make a difference in peoples' lives. Until this day, I have no greater joy than to help people who have disconnected with their authentic selves and have lost the connection between their minds and their bodies because of binge eating behaviors and inactivity. Binge eating affects not just your weight it affects all facets of your life. When someone learns to overcome it, doors all around them begin to open.

What is wrong with willpower?

For many, food is the way to cope with all of the negative situations they deal with on a daily basis. We are conditioned by popular culture that turning to eating is the solution to our problems. Willpower does not work by itself. You need a strong commitment along with a strategy to rid yourself of food addiction and attain freedom. Additionally, you need the decision to change. Eliminating limiting beliefs like "I'm not good enough" or "I've never succeeded before so it's just not going to happen for me" is an important step along the way. Doubt is a barrier. Certainty is what must be created to make this change happen. You can make this happen. This problem is fixable.

It's very difficult to change a behavior when it's habitual and we don't even know what is causing the behavior. We can be triggered constantly simply by driving by certain restaurants or seeing billboard advertisements. In order to create a new pattern you have to become aware of unconscious processes that caused your maladaptive patterns. You can interrupt the old pattern to get a new pattern. You will learn to interrupt the patterns that are keeping you from living your ultimate life.

There is great pleasure in taking control. In order to take back control you must raise your standards, change your beliefs, and adopt strategies for change. Then, you can reinforce and repeat to sustain change for physical freedom, higher levels of energy, increased strength, and improved confidence. You are the one who has to make the decision and this book will guide you to obtain a whole new level and an entirely new life.

What Will It Take to be Free from Binge Eating?

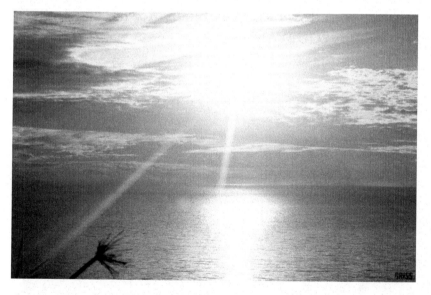

What does it take for you to be free? You are in charge of your body and your mind and your emotions. Want is not enough...it has to be a must. The first stage in your transformation process is to make change a *must*.

By the end of this book, you will be clear about how exactly to master your body and your emotions for a lifestyle transformation. You will be shown the path to freedom from food addiction. In this book, you will learn that you absolutely can stop binge eating behaviors for life. You are about to uncover evidence-based techniques and information that will take you out of your uphill battle with food, help you become unstuck, and lead you on a journey to an amazing life.

If you have tried to stop the endless cycle with food, and you are at a point of hopelessness, you are *not* alone in this struggle. You are about to discover the reasons you are overeating and feeling out of control. You will learn evidence-based solutions to get you out of what seems to be an endless cycle. Today you will learn how to eliminate binge eating behaviors from your life once and for all. Congratulations on your journey to uncover the techniques to get you to THE BODY AND LIFE YOU WANT.

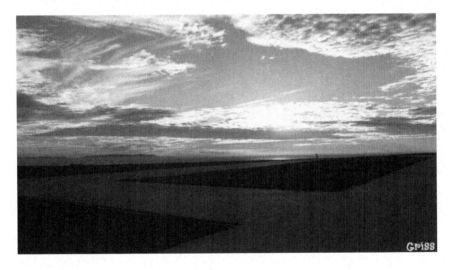

Part I
Getting Started

Chapter One

You Can Say Goodbye to Binge Eating

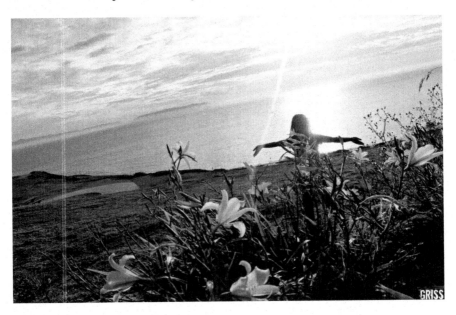

The Facts

Binge eating involves consuming a large amount of food in a discrete time period-typically one to two hours. During a binge eating episode, there's a sense of lack of control once a person begins to eat that they simply cannot stop. During a binge eating episode, there is also a feeling of being disconnected. A large portion of our obese population do suffer from Binge Eating Disorder (BED). It's characteristic of most people that are in the morbid obesity or obesity range. Obesity is a chronic and treatable issue. It is one of the top three *preventable* causes of death.

Interestingly, dieting is common with binge eaters. They spend half of their lives dieting (restricting food). Those who are the most obese typically have a history of dieting a.k.a. food restriction.

It is the addictive-type nature that characterizes Binge Eating Disorder. Like drug addiction, food addiction involves compulsive behaviors as well as neurotransmitters in the brain being affected as a result of the behavior. Food addiction can be a tricky issue to treat since you can't quit eating as people quit drugs. You are forced to deal with food in order to survive. Compulsive overeating is heavy on the hearts of many people because it impacts quality of life. Food addiction and compulsive overeating can cause destruction as it can result in loss of time with loved ones among numerous other consequences.

Food addiction is very real. Certain foods, just like opiates, trigger the same areas of the brain as drugs. Fatty, sugary, and salty foods trigger dopamine release in the pleasure centers of the brain just like crack cocaine or heroin. We know that there is a great deal of pleasure that comes from eating high carbohydrate/high sugar content foods. These type of foods release dopamine (a feel-good chemical) in the brain. Eating foods high in sugar or carbohydrates is a pleasure-seeking behavior. Activation in the reward pathway in the brain tells a person to repeat what they just did to get that reward. So if an activity results in in activation of the reward pathway in the brain, a person is likely to seek to consume rewards such as eating sweets/carbohydrates again and again. Research now shows that junk food is as dangerous as smoking. Just like drugs and alcohol, people use food to comfort years of pain.

The food industry has one goal and that is to make food that is irresistible. They are trying to increase the profit from the food you consume. These companies rely on science to understand how we are attracted to food and how they can make their food attractive to us. The food industry researches the taste receptors on our tongue and the neurochemical reaction in our brain. What is the point of this research? The point is to make you not be able to eat just one.

There is a science behind processed foods. Math and science, and regression analysis perfect the amounts of fat, sugar, and salts that are placed in foods. Food engineering involves chemistry, physics, and biology. Food engineers are able to find ways of enhancing cheese flavor without cheese. Preservatives and ingredients act as flavor enhancers to trick the brain that it's something it's not. They can simulate taste without it being real. As a result, the cost of developing cheese-flavored products and countless other processed products can be reduced significantly.

Food processing industry rests on three pillars: fat, sugar, and salt. These ingredients are what makes food palatable (it's what makes food taste good). Foods that are high in fat, salt, and sugar are the palatable foods. Highly palatable foods can be addictive. One spoonful lights up the brain in clinical trials. Fortunately, there are evidence-based techniques that can help you decrease and eventually eliminate bingeing on these processed palatable foods.

Chapter Two

Self-Sabotaging and the Power of Choice

Why Have You Been Sabotaging Yourself?

Here are some common causes of binge eating:

Emotion: Overeating to celebrate or overeating as a coping mechanism to soothe suffering, loneliness, loss or fears.

Feeling Deprived: You feel deprived of the foods which you enjoy and this leaves you craving for them even more. During certain points in your life you could be engaging in restrictive dieting and avoidance of certain groups of foods. Most people who binge eat have a history of restrictive dieting. Unfortunately, the foods being avoided are abundantly available and availability of foods are powerful eating stimuli. As a result, the restricter often breaks the intended "plan" and eats a "forbidden" food which triggers a binge. Food restriction is one of the biggest psychological and physiological triggers for a binge eating episode.

Stressed or Overwhelmed: Stressful circumstances with work, health problems, finances, relationships, traffic, etc. can set you up for the perfect storm for a binge.

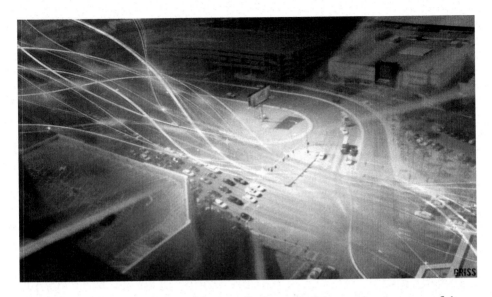

Habit: Binge eating could simply be a habit you've engaged in for so long that it is your top "go-to" no matter what the circumstance. Binge eating for you then is simply habitual. Habit is a likely cause when individuals have grown up around or have had binge eating modeled for them by others.

Tiredness: You are putting up with so much in your life that this is constantly taking away from your sleep time and draining your energy. When your energy level is low, you may look for food to pick you up. It has been shown that tiredness dysregulates hormones in the body and can trigger binges.

Seeking Love and Comfort: You may turn to food when you're really needing love and comfort. Lack of appreciation and/or discouraging remarks by others can leave you feeling down and lonely. If you fit in this category, you tend to turn towards food to find consolation.

Rewards: If you eat to reward yourself, you can relate to a situation where you've worked yourself into the ground one week and you became excited to reward that hard work with food. All diets work in the short-term. The real trick is to maintain those changes. Let's say you lose all the weight you want to lose. How do you maintain it? You don't go to IHOP to celebrate. Instead, you schedule a three-day get away, spa day, or a concert.

Seeking Acceptance: If you eat to feel acceptance, you eat food you wouldn't eat if you were alone.

Boredom: Boredom is a major cause for binge eating. Simply being under-stimulated mentally can trigger the need to seek out spikes in feel-good chemicals in the brain and engage in an activity. In this case, binge eating is the maladaptive activity.

Procrastination: If you eat to procrastinate, then you constantly go to the kitchen to eat to avoid working on whatever needs to get done. You put your work off while you overindulge with snacks.

Body Image Issues: If your focus is on the things which you feel are "wrong" with your body one of your causes for binge eating may be body image issues. One of the reasons people are unable to overcome binge eating triggers is the inability to accept one's body.

Are you physically hungry? Or are you engaging to combat a difficult emotion or are you eating to combat boredom or for some other reason? We will address these questions later on.

The Power of Choice

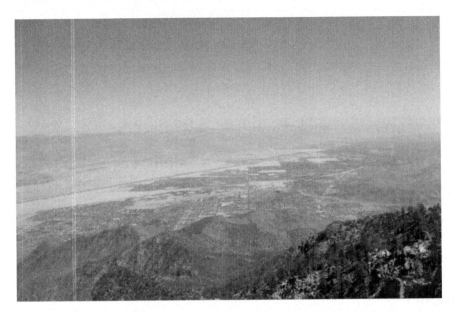

We are happy when we are making progress. We are happiest when we believe statements and affirm statements to ourselves like "I don't need to wait for perfection," "I choose to get fit," "I choose to walk," and "I'm doing it now." You don't need to find the perfect trainer or take all month searching on the internet to find the perfect meal delivery service. Get yourself in a new state. Affirm to yourself that you are changing now. You can change your life remarkably fast with the right choices and the right affirmations to yourself.

People vary in their readiness to change. Prochaska's stages of change include: Pre-contemplation-you haven't even thought about changing; Contemplation-you're aware you might want to change but you're ambivalent because it may be difficult; Preparation-you have a plan and you're about ready to get started; Action-you implement the plan; Maintenance-you sustain change by repeating the behaviors consistently.

Everyone wants a better life but something often gets in the way. Whether it's turning around our finances, or turning around a relationship, or attaining a better body, something gets in the way of progress. Setting out on a new change usually comes because something clicked. Something happened to shift your perception. You break out of the old irrational thinking patterns and you start to make the shift that creates the life you want. When you come up with a new perception you get a new action that, in turn, creates a new result.

What is the power you have in this moment that can change anything? The power of choice. We can't control the events or circumstances but we can choose the meaning we give our circumstances, our perception, and whether or not we will move forward. How is your life better today because of a decision you made years ago?

That decision has affected so much of your life: what you earn, how you feel about yourself, who you have in your life, etc. If you don't like what you have in your life... change it. If you want to change anything in your life then change it. If you want a new life you have to make new decisions. Little decisions like what you eat in the morning and whether or not you have your snack can all add up and create a result you either want, tolerate, or hate. Maybe it's time to change your body. Maybe it's time to change your energy level. Maybe it's time to change your state of health. Whatever it is, a new life comes from new choices but they must be conscious choices. When you make decisions consciously about what to do and how you will do it, you focus on it with conscious intent.

You get to choose the meaning of anything. For example, you can have a difficult time planning meals out and decide to quit or you can alternatively tell yourself you're going to turn your health around and find a way. Whether this is the end or the beginning...it is up to you to decide. Little choices start to affect your entire life. Focus immediately on a solution. Put all of your intention and focus into turning your body (and ultimately your life) around. Breakthroughs start to happen when you decide to change and you shift your focus concentrating solely on *solution*.

What keeps you overweight? You're probably being rewarded. Whatever gets rewarded gets reinforced. You have to believe having a better body and improved health is more pleasurable than overeating and being inactive...period. If you want to make a breakthrough, go through these steps:

Step 1: *See it as it is...not worse.* No matter what you've been through, if you're in a crisis see it as it is but don't see it as worse. You can't make it so horrific that you just give up. When you start thinking there's no future you go into a place of learned helplessness and that's when people get into binge eating, binge drinking, and depression. See it as it is, but don't see it worse than it is so you have no reason to change.

Step 2: *Get to the Truth.* If you are in denial about how much you've tried to lose weight then get to the truth. Start journaling all of the food that you eat throughout the day as well as your activity engagement. The truth is often uncomfortable. It doesn't feel good but we have to get to the truth to change.

Step 3: *Get yourself a vision you want.* You will need something to go for to give you the psychological fuel to move forward. You already know you don't want an overweight body or poor health or low energy levels. Get a vision for what you *do* want. Visualization is used by Olympic athletes. Injured athletes are known for running races in their minds when they can't practice. Olympic competitions have been won as a result of practicing this sport psychology technique. Visualize (using all of your senses) how you want to feel, what you want to see in yourself, how you want others to respond to you, how you will experience the world, and what you will look like when you are mentally and physically improved.

Step 4: *Get a strategy.* One of the things I've noticed that CEOs and self-made millionaires have in common is that they have had mentors in their lives guiding them in the direction of their ideal lives. You can have a mentor simply by watching online videos of someone that has something that you want in your life. Ideally, you would meet with your mentor weekly and you would work out a strategy for change together. A mentor typically already went through ups and downs in their business or healthy lifestyle change and ended up right where you want to be in your life.

Step 5: *Get into action.* There's a quote by Zig Ziglar that applies to action. The quote is "You don't have to be great to start but you have to start to be great." It applies to everyone. I cannot stress the importance of speed of implementation enough. Those who simply get up and decide to start a business and just go have an edge over those who stir, and ruminate, and research, and try to perfect their plan, and contemplate some more, and ultimately waste time thinking without acting. Those who simply get up and decide to start a food and exercise regimen have an edge over those who stir, and ruminate, and research, and try to perfect their plan, and contemplate some more, and ultimately waste time thinking without acting. The point is to just *start.*

Chapter Three

How to Deal with Emotions *without* Using Food

What happens when something's bugging you, or hurting you, or making you feel stressed out? How do you identify whether you are emotionally eating or not?

Virtually everyone has had bouts of emotional eating. Emotional eating takes on different forms. We simply fall on different parts of the spectrum of emotional eating and vary with regard to what degree. The degree to which we are emotionally eating can depend on what kind of challenges you are facing, what season it is, and how you currently identify as a person.

Why do we use food? Our culture is inundated with messages to consume. Most of us have grown up being trained to soothe and reward ourselves with food. What do people do with a fussy toddler? They put cookies or goldfish crackers in front of them to calm them. A second grade teacher rewards her class for getting good grades with suckers. A little league coach rewards the team for winning with pizza and soda. The broken-hearted jump into cupcakes after a breakup.

We are soothing emotions with food. We are celebrating and rewarding ourselves with food. When we are stressed, our body craves high carbohydrate/sugary food like chocolate or chips. We must figure out how to manage these emotions so that we don't binge eat. A lot of us think of food as a reward. We tell ourselves that when we get off work we're going to have a bag of chips or ice cream or French fries etc. If we're eating throughout the day it distracts us and tricks us into thinking we're okay. If we eat large amounts of food and we disconnect while eating, and we feel out of control while we are eating, we are actually engaging in binge eating behaviors.

You may be struggling with how to break away from emotional eating. You may want to be successful, and your mind may seem somewhat ready, but you can't break away from going overboard with your eating.

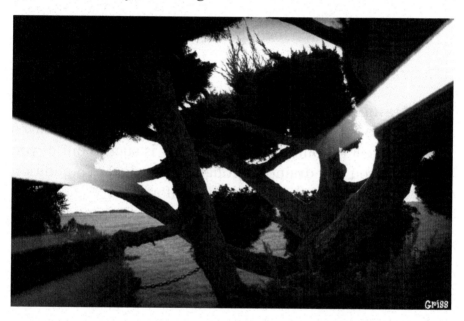

Everyone falls off track with their health at some point. People tend to get thrown off around the issue of emotional eating. When we feel stuck and feel out of control with food, it's critical to look at the issue around the cycle of emotional eating.

There are four main points to look at when it comes to eating to cope with emotions.

1) **Trigger/Emotional Response**-an example of something that triggers an emotion is a breakup or a stressful day at work or even negative thoughts about self.

2) **Cover Up**-cover up includes "numbing out" or disconnecting from the discomfort of the situation with food

3) **False Bliss**-the high that comes from binge eating-but it never lasts.

4) **Hangover**-physical and mental discomfort (the comfort food that people reach for eventually makes you feel uncomfortable-the energy is sucked out of you and you feel drained throughout the day). In addition to the physical pain or discomfort that comes from overeating is the emotional aspect. Guilt and shame from falling off track leads to a new trigger which then continues the cycle of it all.

Getting to the Root of the Problem

Everyone has different triggers and they can be based on insecurities that sometimes stem from childhood. For example, a friend takes a day or two to get back to you and you interpret it as "they don't like me". A trigger can be almost anything. In order to break away from fear and insecurity you can address the issue directly. Overall, you must uncover your fears and insecurities. The way to do just that is by challenging irrational beliefs that are not serving you.

When you find yourself disconnecting while you eat, or when you find yourself feeling an impulse to binge eat, it's important that you are able to identify where you are in the cycle. The more you can bring awareness to your mood state and your feelings before, during, and after you eat the more you can interrupt the cycle. Bring awareness to your mood before, during, and after you overeat or when you have the urge to overeat. On the next page you will be able to work with the mood, thoughts, and food worksheet.

Mood, Thoughts, and Food Log

Mood	Thought	Desired Food
Example: Anxious	I feel like my boss doesn't like my work	Cookies

Filling out this worksheet (or journaling your thoughts and feelings) when you have the urge to binge eat can help you bring unconscious processes to the surface and eventually get you out of the old pattern.

Cravings Worksheet

Detect whether you are emotionally eating or not and be aware of your unconscious and conscious processes. When you're constantly aware of your thoughts it helps because thoughts affect emotions and thoughts create actions. Is your body hungry for nutrients? Are you craving chips and chocolate or maybe you're craving a hug or a vacation to de-stress.

Food Craving	Actual Craving	Way to Cope
Example: Tacos	Relief from stress at work	Schedule self-care time
Example: Donuts	Connectedness	Schedule lunch with old friend

Vulnerability is an important part of recovery in any realm. Don't be afraid to be transparent about what you're going through. Share it with another person that you trust. Say what's in your heart and in your mind.

Fully experience the emotion rather than stuffing it. It's not the easiest thing to do but if we become more aware of our emotions and actions it makes us stronger and more resilient. A study came out that asserted that if we recognize and let ourselves feel and be present with physical pain, it will ease up faster than if we simply try to ignore it. Emotional pain and discomfort are similar to physical pain and discomfort in that same way. If we allow ourselves to be immersed in an emotion (rather than ignoring it) it gives us the opportunity for the negative emotion to alleviate faster.

Constantly check in with yourself. You and others around you have given yourself labels. For example, "I am the caretaker of the entire family" or "I am the weak one in the family" or "I am the scapegoat" or "I am the overachiever so I can't disappoint." Take a look at the roles you are trying to fill and see how authentic they are to you and what you want.

Emotion regulation involves the things you do on a regular basis to regulate your emotions. There are things we do that dysregulate us as well as regulate us. Over-sleeping (which is also known as hypersomnia) is dysregulating. Over-sleeping is a maladaptive way to "check out" so it is not recommended by mental health professionals. Under-sleeping is even more dysregulating, resulting in negative mood and hormone dysregulation that will trigger a binge.

In evidence-based therapies, mental health professionals talk about the importance of increasing one's pleasurable activities to better regulate negative emotions (like sadness, anger, and frustration) and prevent maladaptive behaviors. *Most people who binge eat could use an increase in their pleasurable activities.* Pleasurable activities are things you love to do and they may be things you used to love to do but binge eating has gotten in the way either by making you feel self-conscious, physically weak, isolative, and/or depressed. Engaging in pleasurable activities is a positive distraction away from engaging in binge eating behaviors. If you are a person who enjoys tennis, your recommendation would be to increase the time that you're hitting the ball.

Positive distractions like playing your favorite sport, or listening to music, getting a massage, or reading a book are doubly rewarding because they take away the bad and give us something good. A patient spent years of her life going to weight loss camps, doing extreme juice diets and finally realized her binge eating was about emotions. Using food to cope is like using a hammer when you really need a screwdriver. It's also like a mechanic switching parts out instead of finding the cause of the problem.

No amount of candy, French fries, or tacos can satisfy you more than temporarily. But why can't you stop? More than likely it's some emotional need that we're trying to resolve or satisfy. For instance, you don't like working a 9 to 5 because you told yourself you would be self-employed by now or you feel alone even within your relationship. During evaluation of a client, many times I stumble upon a relationship issue. For example, a client needs to refine boundary setting skills other coping skills. Once they do this, they nullify the need to cope with anything using food.

There are many recommendations out there as far as coping with emotional eating. They tend to be things that take place after the fact that involve distraction tools. However, it is important to be preventative, preemptive, and proactive in our behaviors such as scheduling the positive distraction time (doing something you are stimulated by) or self-care time (doing something nice for yourself) *before* you are already in an isolative, stressed, or depressed state.

Chapter Four

Interpersonal Effectiveness

In clinical practice, we assess for (not only patterns of behavior and in what contexts clients eat) but we also identify what sets them off or what "triggers" them. Examples of triggers could be interactions with a spouse, intrusive family members, and negative co-workers. More than likely, we can't avoid these people in totality. However, you may be engaging in binge eating as an avoidance mechanisms. Not being present by binge eating is an avoidance mechanism to avoid connecting with partner or someone else around you. Extra weight as well as binge eating can act as an unconscious barrier between you and those close to you. In a conscious relationship it's important to close these exits.

We can figure out a way to deal with those around us and identify what to do when they trigger us. Many times, we're indulging in food because it's the one thing we feel we have to give back to ourselves. When we constantly give and tend to others' needs we are left at the end of the day feeling depleted and it feels like there is nothing for ourselves...except for food. We can find ourselves giving to others more than we receive leaving us to fill the void by eating.

Emotional connection and physiology can play a role in helping to curb food cravings. It is possible that the culprit behind over-snacking could be negative feelings about oneself or a lost physical or emotional connection with one's partner. Therefore, there is the potential that a renewed intimate connection could help decrease over-snacking behaviors.

The key is to engage in alternative pleasurable behaviors. When you engage in alternative pleasurable behaviors, you are also forming new habits and, when there is pleasure involved, the brain will begin to seek more of the behavior thus creating more of these behaviors rather than overeating behaviors.

Boundaries for Interpersonal Effectiveness

A boundary is something that sets limits or bounds. With personal boundaries, the focus is on making interactions comfortable so that people can experience closeness. Boundaries allow us to be assertive without being offensive and to experience other people without being offended. Boundaries allow us to protect ourselves physically, sexually, emotionally, and intellectually from the unwanted intrusions of others. They also allow us to contain ourselves so that we behave in a way that doesn't offend others.

Boundaries can help us avoid behaving too passively or passive aggressively. Setting a protective boundary is considered an act of self-acceptance. Learning to set personal boundaries leads to respectful intimacy and leads to better sense of self. Most people feel wounded from past experiences. As a result, and because of a lack of acceptance of ourselves, we fear being disliked or dismissed or being disapproved of, or that others will know the worst about ourselves. Then we go too far with our giving and we give in too easily to others' requests. Boundaries help us get back to balance within a relationship.

As we practice boundaries we are on the way to self-acceptance which gradually helps us believe that we are lovable.

Take inventory of the relationships in your life. Without judging, notice what relationships you are giving more than receiving. Ask yourself if you need to change the dynamics of the relationships. Spending more time with people who give back can help you to feel less depleted. Also, it is possible to shift the dynamics within your relationships by saying no more often (this is an example of a boundary) or asking for what you need more often.

In any kind of relationship (romantic, family, or friendship) you can assess priorities so that that it is balanced. These priorities are:

1) **Getting What You Want** (requesting what you want or refusing someone else's request)

Refusing someone's request:

Saying no to what you don't want can be difficult because you are feeling guilty or worried that you will be rejected. When a person is afraid to disappoint someone it can result in resentment or passive aggressive behaviors on their part thus destroying authenticity and relationships. If you are angry and you are pretending that you are not you might be presenting as passive aggressive. For example, giving the silent treatment is just as passive aggressive as "fine you go out with the boys and I'll just sit here all by myself." Passive aggressiveness can be damaging to a relationship. No one gets what they want all the time and that's okay. Saying no is not selfish...it is oftentimes necessary for the health of you and your relationship.

To get what you want in a relationship use the acronym DEARMAN:

D-Describe the situation, E-Express how you feel, A-Ask for what you want, R-Reinforce the other person (I appreciate you being interested), M-Mindful-stick with present not past issues, A-Appear confident (make eye contact and be self-assured), and finally N-Negotiate-give something up (but not too much) and compromise.

2) **Maintaining or Building the Relationship** (Balance: knowing when to let things go for the sake of the relationship and when to not). Don't try to guess what someone wants...ask them. Workable compromise involves offering to compromise with something. It's never healthy to compromise core issues-things you would have to change about yourself so you're no longer authentic to what you feel strongly about.

3) **Self-Respect** (We have values that we're sticking to and our identity is in place).

Part II

Altering Thoughts and Behaviors for the Body You Want

Chapter Five

Set goals like a Champion

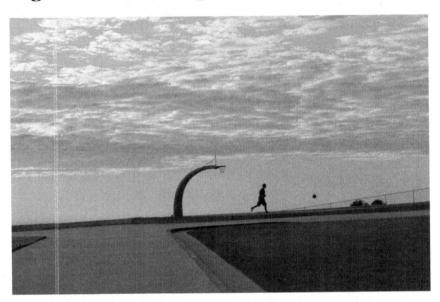

We've all set New Year's goals. What makes resolutions fail? Many people fall victim to a concept called learned helplessness. They repeat the messages that keep them down like "I can't do it," "I've tried so many times," "I've never done it before," or "I know it's not going to work this time."

Is there a limit to how good you can look and feel? The answer is no...and if you previously held this belief it was a lie. Your limiting beliefs (like the ones previously stated) can be broken and no matter what has happened previously you can get to your next level.

What actually makes goals work? Studies show that people who write their goals down accomplish their goals more often than those who do not. Journal what your health might be like, what your lifestyle will be like, how much you will be playing with your child outside, how many sports you will play, how many outdoor adventure trips you will take when you accomplish your goal. A very important realization for you is this... you probably don't have enough goals now. You might have some goals. Even someone who is not into personal development may say they have goals. If you think that you have goals right now, you may actually not have solid goals.

Goal Setting in Action

Your goals have costs. Every meaningful goal has a cost. You're not going to create a relationship without cost. You're not going to build a business without cost (time or money cost or time away from friends and family). You have to be okay with costs. You can't pay someone to do your push-ups for you or eat your meals for you. You are going to sacrifice to get the behaviors and ultimately the body you want.

Setting a clear and solid goal helps you focus on relevant activities that will get you there as opposed to trying to do everything and not fully accomplishing much. There's a big difference between *hoping* you achieve goals and *expecting* that you will achieve your goals.

It's imperative that you know what you want and how you are going to achieve it. You need a compelling vision so it keeps you going through the ups and downs. Visions work because there's a challenge and challenges keep you engaged. When you're committed you're not taking no for an answer; you're not taking the easy way out; you're willing to do whatever it takes. Move on to the next milestone as you get closer and closer to your vision. Then see yourself successfully stepping up to that ultimate vision and achieving it.

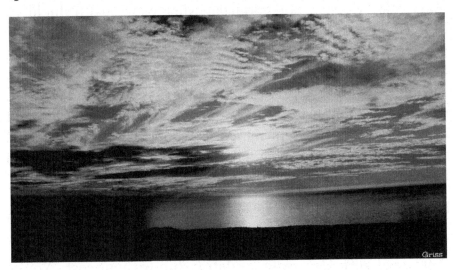

Experiment:

Imagine yourself hoping that you will live a healthy lifestyle. Close your eyes and picture yourself hoping you will feel the way you will feel and breathe how you breathe when you hope, think "I really hope I will accomplish my goal" "I hope I will be at my peak health state", "I hope that I get the body I want", "I hope, I hope, I hope".

Now, close your eyes and imagine yourself expecting that you *will* achieve the body, health and energy you want. Breathe how you breathe when you expect yourself to accomplish that goal. Feel yourself in your new body and tell yourself "I expect to achieve my goal", "I will have the body I want", "I will feel amazing."

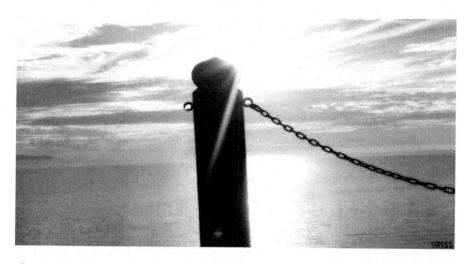

If you went through this exercise, you should have felt a difference between how you feel when you have a vague goal (simply hoping for achievement) and how you feel when you are actually *expecting a change.*

A vague desire of wanting something better is not going to be enough. For example, "I wish my business was earning twice as much," or "I wish I wasn't so negative," or "I wish my health was better." You can start there, but you can't stay there, not if you want to get to your goal. If it's not solid and you don't believe it, it's not going to get realized; it will just remain in fantasy land. The goal must be inspiring in order to sustain the costs that it takes to achieve the goal. You can start to affirm to yourself "I'm going to look different in my photos," "I'm going to have more options with romantic partners," "I'm going to have more energy," "I'm going to be more confident at work which will increase my earning potential."

There are five points that demonstrate a proper goal:

1) Goal needs to be specific –The better clarity you have about what you want, the more your behaviors will follow those cognitions.   Clarification is critically important; specificity is critical.

2) Size of goal should be big and compelling-The goal should inspire you.

3) Written down –A goal can easily be too vague if it's only in your head. Write your goal down so you can refer back to it during the process and after you achieve it.

4) Review goal every day like clockwork -Look at it every day until it's accomplished. So it's always top of mind. If it's a goal that takes a month or five months or a year, writing it down and stuffing it in your drawer is detrimental.

5) Goal should be aligned with your values- Know your life purpose.

Every day, close your eyes, breathe deeply into your center and imagine yourself at your peak. If you're trying to master something like your weight or your fitness level, there will be a major mental component involved. Engineer your environment to be successful with your goal. Construct a lifestyle that's devoted to both physical and mental components of peak performance now that this is your top priority and focus. Getting to your goal should be enjoyable. In order for you to maintain permanent change the process needs to be enjoyable.

Goals matter...There has been a ton of research on the goals that motivate and the ones that don't. The goals that matter and motivate behavior change are hard and specific. "Do Your Best" goals do not motivate. For example, "I'm going to try to organize my house," or "I'm going to be a nicer person." In order to have goals with the outcome of success, we sequence them; we break them down. For instance, a long term goal is to drop three dress sizes. Then we break it up by setting a goal every day and setting a goal every week. You add that up and you've got that goal accomplished.

Chapter Six

All-or-Nothing Thinking and Dealing with Adversity

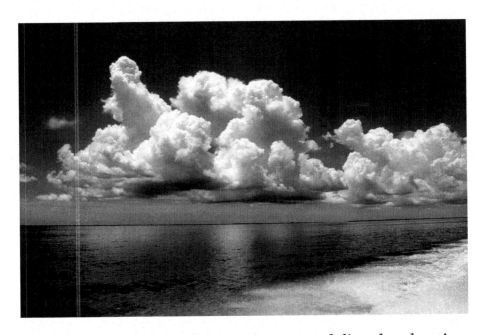

Food-shaming can result in an increase of disordered eating patterns. Food shaming (telling yourself that a particular food is good or bad) comes from black and white thinking (also known as dichotomous thinking). Black and white thinking is all-or-nothing thinking and it sets you up for failure. An example of this type of thinking could be "Birthday cake is bad so I can never eat it" or "Carbs are bad so if I eat them, I'm bad."

Ten plus years ago, most personal trainers would ask their clients to strictly adhere to a meal plan and would provide a list of off-limit foods. We don't see this type of restriction as much anymore because we know that it can be dangerous for clients that have a history of binge eating or restricting behaviors resulting from all-or-nothing/black-or-white cognitions. If a trainer or a dietitian told you that a particular food is bad or off limits you may be tempted to restrict and deny yourself that food. Then, when you eventually give in to eating that food you had been depriving yourself of you eat much more of it because you think you'll never get it again. You may also become racked with guilt so you need more of it to numb out and to satisfy.

Today, fitness trainers and dietitians are more educated about the risk of food-shaming and know that when people feel shamed by eating certain foods they will have an all or nothing attitude and be set up for failure. They think "I blew today so the rest of the day I'm going to eat whatever I want." If all foods are allowed, then there is no shame in working favorite foods into a caloric allotment or meal plan whether it's to lose or to maintain weight.

What to do about Adversity

I have a message I want to share with you about adversity. There are many times in life when circumstances will hit you hard and you will not know what to do. Maybe something happens to your health, or your partner breaks up with you, or someone that you love dies. What will you do?

You're floating along and things are going well. You're making money or your relationship is going great (or you think it's going great)...and sure enough you get hit by adversity-something outside of your control. You are hit hard. When events like this happen, most people become stressed, anxious, and disabled by uncertainty.

It is right in that moment you have to decide what you're going to do.

There are two decisions you can make in the moment. One, you can be a victim of the situation-you can give up hope and just give up on life. You can sit around, eat food, watch TV, and find every distraction to disconnect from the pain or discomfort. Then you can inevitably find yourself a year from that point looking the same way and feeling the same way.

The other option (which in my opinion is the only option) is to use what is given to you. See it as something that will make you stronger. I'm going to give you an example of a bodybuilder. In order to build muscle he has to work-out to "failure" until the point that he cannot complete one more lift. After the reparative process, he builds more muscle tissue and becomes even stronger because of that "failure."

The best CEOs have built bigger companies after going through bankruptcy. Life doesn't happen to you. Life happens for you. If you really believe that, you can free yourself up in so many ways. Find the empowering meaning. We know from studies that people who get through pain, suffering, and adversity successfully are the people who find *purpose in their suffering*.

The only thing you can do is take action. Ask yourself what's great about this? How can I learn from this? How can I grow from this? How can I turn this around? How can I use this experience and teach others and serve others in some way?

Focus on what people are good at, what you are good at, and what you can do to make things better. Problems are a real part of life and they cannot simply be ignored. However, obstacles can be challenged and reframed as opportunities for growth. If you can change the way you look at your challenges, you can give yourself a different perspective.

Sometimes your worst days can be your best days because those days make you motivated to act. They help you to teach and inspire others simply because you got through something... simply because you experienced it and overcame it.

You can use whatever life has given you to make yourself stronger and allow those experiences to make you grow. If you're going through some adversity in life, and you apply some of my message about adversity, it can make you look at what you're going through differently and you can use it as your motivation to take action so you can achieve more out of life.

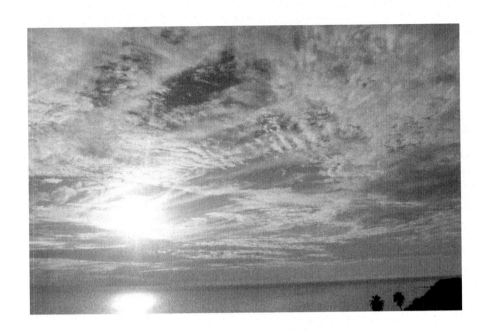

Chapter Seven

Positive Psychology

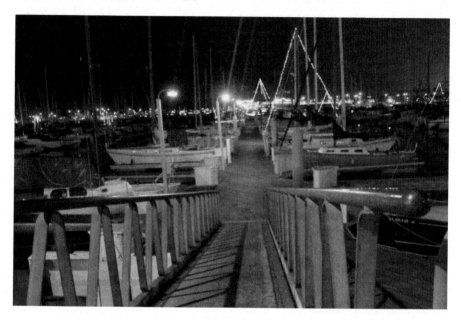

Binge Eating from a Positive Psychology Perspective

Meaning/Purpose, Activity, and Connectedness

When you're at the bottom (stuck inside your own head) how can you come out of it? Change your perspective. Stop isolating. Studies show that isolating makes you feel worse in the long-run. Do something that scares you. You won't know what to expect but it's likely what you need to do to feel healing and feel closer to your true identity. Align your actions and how you spend your time with your mission in life. If your health isn't up to par or your body isn't how you want it, you may be living according to an old blueprint. At some point, we follow that blueprint or we fight it. There can be conflict between what you desire most and what you believe you can do according to the story you give your life. Write your old story...include limiting beliefs like "I'm not good-looking enough," "No one cares what I have to say," "I can never have the body I want," "I will never be successful"... What is stopping you from having everything you've ever wanted? Write your limiting story here with all those limiting beliefs:

_____

_____

_____

_____

_____

_____

_____

_____

_____

_____

_____

_____

_____

_____

_____

_____

What do you want? What do you need? What will you have? What is your new story? Rewrite it:

_____
_____
_____
_____
_____
_____
_____
_____
_____
_____
_____
_____
_____
_____
_____
_____
_____
_____

Sometimes you have to fake it 'til you make it. Sometimes you have to do things that are uncomfortable or that you feel is somewhat inauthentic in order to get into the mindset you need to engage in behaviors that are aligned with your positive identity.

Positive Psychology for Lifestyle Change

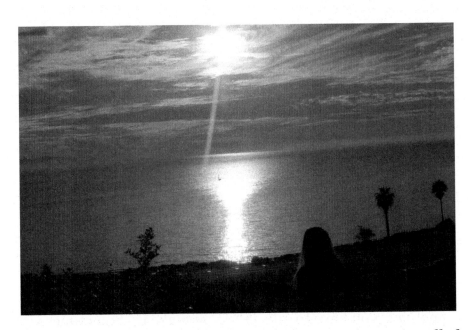

The scientific study of what makes life worth living is called *positive psychology*. Positive psychology leads us to focus on healthy habits. Positive psychologists are interested in talents, passions, and what gets people up in the morning. They focus on things like optimism, character, health, and well-being. Lives can shift dramatically when the focus is on personal strengths such as sense of humor, athletic abilities, work skills, and passions.

What is the relationship of happiness to a life well-lived? Happiness is an indicator but it's not a perfect indicator. Studies show that people function at their best when they fulfill their needs of **pleasure, engagement, relationships, and achievement.**

Life is more than getting rid of problems. Happiness involves something more. According to the research, meaning and purpose are necessary ingredients for happiness. Happiness comes not necessarily from the pursuit of happiness in itself, but from the pursuit of things that makes life worth living. Happiness is a product of our pursuits like the amount of time you spend playing with your kids, the time away for travel, and the amount of time you spend engaging in steps toward your dream career or lifestyle. It has been shown that in order to feel truly happy one needs a sense of purpose and meaning. Purpose and meaning can be found in friends and family, travel, activity/sports, studies, volunteering, and work.

People are always looking for the shortcuts, the "Seven Easy Steps" and the easy formula for feeling good. Studies show that you have to work at it. Happiness comes from small things that you do over and over again that result in building connections with people or building the body you want or the energy level you want. These behaviors will be repeated when there is reinforcement. A shy person can force themselves to be chatty and it pays off. A person that usually lays around can force themselves to be an avid exerciser if it pays off. In order to receive the payoff, one must be consistent.

We are happiest when we are in an environment in which excellence is celebrated, recognized, and nurtured. Affirmations plus action equals results. Happiness is not a selfish concern. It has benefits for those around you. According to the research, happy people are more successful at school and more successful at work. They also have better relationships and they live longer.

Happiness contributes to success. We know that most people are resilient. Strengths of people matter. Perseverance predicts success at school, work, and health transformations. Every finding in positive psychology study implicates that other people matter. It's in our relationships that we find our real source of happiness. Isolating because of the way you look or because of your out of control eating behaviors puts you in a position of missing out on one major component of happiness-connectedness. Other people matter-mentors, trainers, coaches. You want mentors that are going to be engaged with you fully. Friends who tell you that you can't are the ones that can't do it themselves.

Good days have common factors according to the studies. In one study, researchers asked people at the end of a day if it was a good day for them. If it was a good day, they had to describe what they did during that day. There were surprising similarities across cultures.

#1 We have good days when we do things we feel *competent* about and we use our skills.

#2 We have good days when we have a sense of *choice* over what we did that day.

#3 We have good days when we feel *connected* to other people.

Automatize mindful eating and fitness habits. People are really good at making excuses to overeat and to not go to the gym. At this moment, you may be "de-conditioned" (a fancy term for being out of shape). You can automatize a workout and you can also automatize balanced eating by forming the behavior and having enough *reasons* and *rewards*.

Be aware of the consequences. When consequences of a behavior are desirable we are more likely to engage in that behavior. When consequences are punitive we'll be less likely to do it. When we go to the gym and we feel like one of the biggest persons there it can be very intimidating and it can feel punitive. If this is a definite barrier, have fitness trainers come to you. If you only like working out alone, there are home regimens and home equipment, and workout videos you can use. If you like being around other people, find a bootcamp, dance class, water aerobics class, kickboxing class, or a hiking meetup group. Minimize the aversiveness of the experience so that there is no longer a barrier.

We already know the risks for poor health-too much salt, excess sugar intake, smoking, overeating, and under-exercising. What are the indicators of positive health? Hopeful and optimistic people have better cardiac health. Those with a sense of meaning and purpose in life are healthier. Health assets include biological assets, psychological assets, and functional assets (e.g. having a job that fits what you're all about). Schedule a place to get in shape, a plan to eat mindfully..make your goals attainable not DYB ("do your best").

Improved Thinking for a Fit Body

We are what we do. Habits matter. The best way to establish a habit is to be aware and monitor it. Say to yourself, "Let me keep track of this." Ask yourself, "What triggers me to eat?", "What are the coping skills that I can use to overcome this?"

Positive psychology supports the idea that reframing helps with sustaining motivation for your goals.

Reframe Example:

Negative Thought: "This hurts"

Reframe: "There is good pain and bad pain...exercise is good pain."

The other part of reframing is focusing on what you have accomplished. For example, what you have accomplished as opposed to how far you have to go. You may not have lost any body fat the first few days, but you can focus on what you have accomplished with regard to your eating and physical activity the last few days. This is a positive reframe. Studies show that people can be more effective with their weight loss goals if they focus on their behavioral accomplishments (i.e. showing up for a workout) rather than the outcome alone (i.e. weight, pant size).

Flow

There is a psychological notion known as *flow*. Flow is happening for you when time flies and you are invigorated in whatever activity in which you are engaged. Research into flow shows that it is invigorating in its aftermath as well. Everyone can find flow. Flow can be experienced when you are fully immersed in reading, or art, or in a game, or watching a game, or in a project you are excited about completing, or playing your favorite sport, or writing a song etc. When you are in flow, you look up and say "Wow I've been doing this for hours and I haven't had any urges to order food or go to the kitchen."

Peak-end Theory

End your balanced eating and/or physically active day on a high note. Peak-end theory says we need high peaks at the end so you'll repeat the behaviors on future days. Restriction of enjoyment is your enemy when you are letting go of binge eating. Reward is your best friend. What can you end the day with to reward yourself other than food?

1. _____

2. _____

3. _____

4. _____

5. _____

Connectedness, physical activity, and purpose and meaning are the main ingredients for happiness. When we are truly happy, there is less of a need for self-sabotaging behaviors like binge eating.

Discover what gives you a sense of self-worth or mastery. Do something on a regular basis that makes you feel purpose, engage in activities that are physical, and be with others that make you feel connected. Then, reward yourself at the end of the day with something that complements your new healthy lifestyle so you'll be sure to want to repeat!

Chapter Eight

Mindfulness

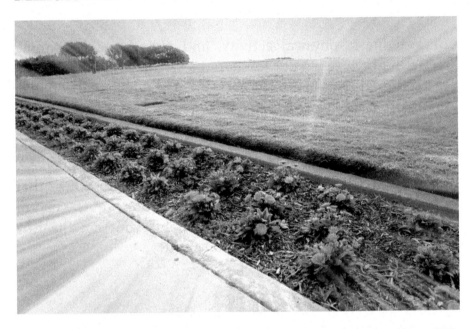

Mindfulness involves a shift in the way you pay attention. We all have numerous thoughts every minute. These thoughts can lead to anxiety, tension, and depression. Mindfulness helps us to lower our stress level and improve mood. It helps us to deepen our connection with ourselves. Mindfulness is the concept of being fully present in each moment. Mindfulness means paying attention on purpose in the present moment non-judgmentally. It is attending to things we might habitually ignore. It requires a focus on the here and now.

When we are practicing mindfulness, we radically accept anything that comes into our thoughts and into our environment. With mindfulness, we look at thoughts objectively when they come up, we look at thoughts from a distance, and we look at them with curiosity rather than judgment.

Can you remember a time when you were total engaged in an activity? Every part of your being was focused on being in the moment. Maybe you experienced it surfing a wave or watching a sunset. Artists know mindfulness when they are absorbed by the moment during creation of art. The keys to fulfillment lie in the state of our minds and the quality of our consciousness.

There are three components to mindfulness. First, our attention is held on purpose. Mindfulness involves the conscious and deliberate direction of our awareness. This is the opposite of auto pilot. When we are on auto pilot there is endless chatter in our minds. Mindfulness allows us to wake up out of auto pilot. It allows us to hold attention where we consciously choose. The second component of mindfulness is that we are immersed in the present moment. Without mindfulness, we get caught up in the past and the future. Mindful attention is completely engaged in the present moment experience-the here and the now. Third, when we practice mindfulness our attention is held non-judgmentally. We are aiming not to control our thoughts in any way. We simply aim to pay attention to our experiences without judging, labeling, or making stories about them in any way.

Eating compulsively takes us away from the present moment. We disconnect and we might miss out on something great. Mindfulness lets us be observers of thoughts that enter and we can imagine them floating away. It allows us to pay attention and refine our ability to pay attention. We are only alive in one moment and that is this moment. Mindfulness-based training is a deep engagement with the vitality of the moment.

It helps us to relieve stress which has a powerful effect on the body.

Mindfulness can be expressed in many types of ways. Meditation is a common form of mindfulness. Yoga is another form of mindfulness. Yoga is an optimal way of connecting mind and body. An added bonus of yoga is that it helps those with body image issues become more one with their bodies and it helps them gain a better acceptance of their bodies. For this reason, yoga is now offered in many eating disorder programs.

Mindfulness can take other forms like taking a walk. A mindful walk would involve being aware of the scenery. Notice the colors, noticing the scents, feeling the air hitting your face. Using all of your senses is an important component of mindfulness because it helps you become completely present. Mindfulness can be practiced anywhere, in any activity, and it can take many forms. It can be in the form of therapy known as Mindfulness-based therapy. It can be practiced while playing a sport, or reading a book, or listening to a guided imagery, or talking to your partner, or listening to music. This list is by no means exhaustive.

You are fully engaged in the moment when you are practicing mindfulness. You are paying attention to everything in the moment with all of your senses. You are fully present and immersed in the activity. Mindfulness techniques can have a powerful effect on your mood, your state of mind, stress reduction, and it can be used as a coping skill when you are feeling triggered to binge eat. *Remember mindfulness for your go-to list when you are feeling the urge to binge eat.*

Program Your Mind to Start Eating Mindfully

If binge eating has been a problem for you, then your mind is focused on stopping binge eating. However, in order to change this pattern, you must focus on the solution-which is mindful eating. Mindful eating is a practice which focuses on solution rather than the problem. You will learn how to eat mindfully later on in this book.

Part III

Action Plan for Results

Chapter 9

The Regimen for Jumpstarting Your Day

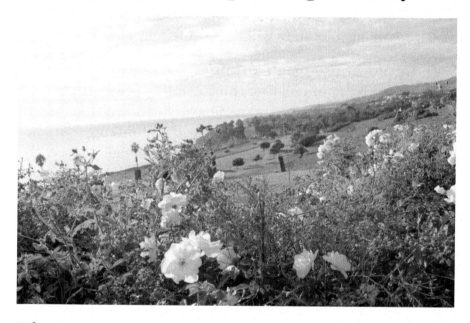

What can you do to make sure you have a successful day? How you start the day is how you end the day. Right when you get out of bed you want to make sure you have a process to take care of yourself mentally, emotionally, and physically throughout the day. A visual representation in your bedroom or somewhere in your home of your routine is helpful.

Most people live their lives reacting to the demands of everyone else. They wake up and they responds to everyone else (check their emails). They don't give themselves the time to nurture and improve the relationship with self. Having a morning regimen can put you in the state to be at your best.

The first thing in the morning you begin to engage in a regimen that will put you in your best mindset. You want to make sure you take care of yourself physically, emotionally and mentally to make sure you're at your best. You don't hope, you demand it. Today is going to be inevitable. You put yourself in the state it takes to win. You don't hope that you're going to make the right decisions to care for yourself like eating right, working out, and preventing burnout. By the end of your regimen your state will be heightened.

1) **Smile-non-verbalizations**... After waking up, as you're lying in bed first thing...smile. See your day as a new opportunity to experience everything life has to offer. Some people start the day thinking "No not another day." Make a conscious choice to see the positive and pick something to look forward to in your day.

2) **Stretch**-As you lay in bed or just after you get out loosen up your muscles wake up your body

3) **Breathe-** Take in several deep belly breaths also known as diaphragmatic breathing. Take the time to take in deep slow diaphragmatic breaths. Inhale and hold. Fully oxygenate your cells and exhale.

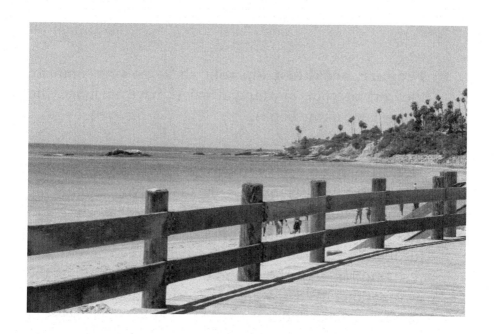

4) **Hydrate-** Your body is desperate for water in the morning. Rehydrate your cells to give yourself everything it needs to be at its best. Alkaline water is recommended. Squeeze organic lemon in your water to make the water more alkalined. Drink two glasses of water right away.

5) **Engage your physiology.** Get moving right away. Get a mini trampoline and use it every single day to get your body awake and alive. Jump up and down...it's a lot of fun. If you don't want a rebounder you can use a jump rope or simply do some jumping jacks in place. There are so many amazing benefits to this process. When you do this you are stimulating your lymphatic system. It helps the toxicity in your body to get flushed out. It's fun and it gives you energy. Start moving your body right away.

6) **Prepare breakfast** Sip your shake as you complete the rest of your morning ritual (I have included the recipe later in the book).

7) **Use Positive Affirmations**-Recondition certain beliefs you want to have to make sure you're mentally strong. Use affirmations like "I'm confident" and "I'm an athletic person." Use phrases that put you in your ideal state. Match your nonverbal to the content and put emotion into the content. Get excited about the affirmations "What I choose to do today is going to shape my today and tomorrow!" , "I enjoy the process of creating a fit body!", "Mindful eating is my way of life", and "I will improve every day." Say these affirmations out loud and put feeling behind it. Use your emotions as you're doing it to keep yourself in the right state.

8) **Empowering Questions**-What you focus on you will feel. Thoughts create emotions which create behaviors. Many people live their lives in reaction. You can ask the right questions to control your perspective and focus on what you have control over instead of reacting to the external circumstances of life. Ask yourself these questions aloud. "What am I happy about in my life?"

Take a moment after each question to consider how the answers to these questions make you feel. Ask yourself what you are proud of in your life. Ask yourself what you are grateful for most. Ask yourself who is it that you love. Ask yourself what you are passionate about most. Ask yourself what you are committed to in your life. Ask "What am I excited about in my life right now? " You could say "Today's going to be an amazing day" and "Incredible things are going to happen today." Then list all of the things you are excited about in your day and in your life.

Spend five minutes a day going through these questions and answering them in a positive way. Through this process you will feel excitement and incredible emotions. Take the time each day to give that to yourself.

9) **Focus on vision and purpose**-Visualize and remind yourself of your purpose and how you want your life to play out. Go into your identity, your code of conduct, what your committed to (your values and goals). Visualize your body looking how you want to look and the lifestyle you want to attain.

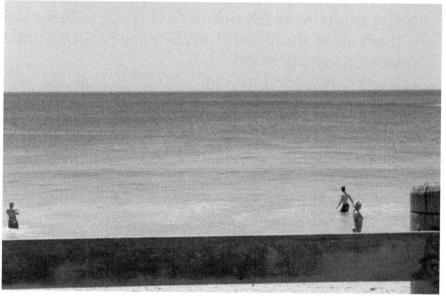

10) **Plan out your day in detail**-You will need a plan of action including an end of the day plan with a result for your body, energy level, the amount of time you spend with people you enjoy etc. Write down actions you need to achieve the end of day result. Plan out your life in detail so you're not simply reacting to life or whatever everyone else has planned for you. Be proactive versus reactive.

11) **Accountability Call**-Each morning, talk with someone about three things you're committed to doing in the day. These are the three things you're going to get done. Next day follow up with friend. If you don't follow through you commit to donate $10 or $20 to charity.

12) **Get ready to work-out.** Working out will give you the strength and high that will help you perform at your best throughout the day.

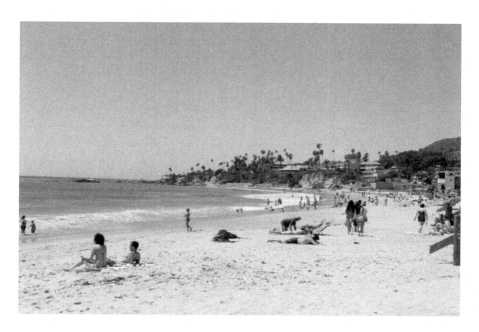

Go-to List

Throughout the rest of your day you most likely will be triggered to overeat. Behavioral modification is a tool we use to change a behavior. We can replace old behaviors with new behaviors. Behavior modification has the potential to be highly adaptive and beneficial from a health and weight loss standpoint. Binge eating is a response to something that is triggering you like stress, boredom, frustration, dissatisfaction etc. Set yourself up for success by creating a go-to list when you are feeling triggered. Instead of giving into self-destructive behaviors (like binge eating) you can access this list. Include things like downloading music, relaxing on the sand, finding a new podcast, getting a chair massage, or relaxing in a sauna or steam room.

Chapter 10

66 Day Challenge

Everything is exciting for a while, a relationship, a diet etc. The secret to sustaining excitement is progress. If we can make progress on a regular basis that's sustaining. Your body is going to change all the time. Progress is not automatic. You have to take control of your life and not just hope like people do when they make a resolution. People make a wish list and they call it a resolution.

Statistics show that January 15th is the cut off when it comes to New Year's resolutions. The majority of people make weight loss resolutions. Ninety-five percent of people who have made a resolution have actually broken the resolution by Jan 15th. The sixty-six day challenge and the tools throughout this book will help you get way beyond and create lasting change in your life. Some people don't even make a resolution so they don't disappoint themselves. The question is what is it that makes us want to make a resolution? The calendar gives us the idea that we can have a fresh start. If you didn't use it effectively, create an experience where on a regular basis you feel like your life is making progress. When you resolve "This is how it's going to be" then you cut off all other possibilities than your commitment.

Ultimately if you're going to change you must raise your standards. You may not get your shoulds (i.e. should stop eating all sugar) but you will get your musts (your standards). When you decide something is a must for you then you make a real resolution and you raise the standard. Have you ever had a standard? Maybe you wanted to quit something one day then something tipped you over and something shifted and you said no more. Is there an area like that in your life? Where you don't go back? When we make something a must it becomes part of our identity. We have to shift how we identify ourselves (You are not a binge eater, you are a person who eats mindfully). We need to stay consistent with how we identify ourselves. Then our behaviors can be aligned with our new identity.

When our identities are out of whack we say things like "I can't do that I'm not that kind of person." When did you come up with this? These types of negative affirmations are based on a set of beliefs that you made a long time ago about what you are capable of and what you will and won't be able to do. No longer accept these limitations. Shift your standards set the bar higher and identify as a person that follows through with progress in some area such as having an ideal body and lifestyle.

We live according to the identity we have for ourselves. It's who you are and you do whatever is required to maintain that identity. Once that becomes your identity that's who you are and that's the ways you live. People who have a fit mentality have rituals...habits they do daily that create more energy, improved mood, and higher self-esteem. They schedule workouts and they feel uncomfortable when they go too long off track. They eat to fuel their bodies.

This is for you...

I'm going to transform my body in the next 66 days. I already see myself as

looking_____

_____

_____and

feeling_____

_____

_____

_____

_____

_____

My reasons for changing

are_____

_____

_____and now it's my standard

to be a person

that_____

_____

_____

_____

_____

_____

_____

_____

_____

What does it take to create lasting change? The first step is like making a resolution, but it is much more than that...it's having a true vision. It needs to be compelling and have the power to pull you. It needs to have something so attractive that it lasts. You will need emotional intensity attached to your vision. You need a strong enough reason that you're going to follow through when the going gets tough. It needs to be so strong that you can push through when challenges come up and when you have no time and you're stressed out. If you have strong enough reasons they can take you through. It must be a compelling vision and you must have strong enough reasons. This way, even if you veer away you can get right back on target to keep making progress.

There's never been a study that says that people can will themselves to lose weight...it's all about habits.

Success results from a series of habits...little things you do consistently that result in amazing things. What kinds of habitual things can you do on a daily basis that will transform your mind body and overall life quality? It doesn't take twenty-eight days (like it is popularly quoted in the media) to break a habit or form a new habit. It actually takes sixty-six days to break an old habit or form a new habit. Exercising every day is a habit. Eating junk food every day is a habit. We can implement more habits that will align us with our goals, dreams and our purpose in life. We can step out of our comfort zone.

If we remain within our comfort zone then we won't grow. In order to achieve anything good we have to step outside which is a very uncomfortable place for most of us. The first sixty-six days require a lot of discipline and after those sixty-six days, behaviors have a significantly better chance at becoming automatic. New dopamine receptors in the brain are then created giving you more of a high when you're active. You will start to feel irritable and you won't feel right when you miss a workout or you overeat.

Reinforce yourself when you stay on track for the most part and avoid self-shaming as well as other people who are critical. Find a supportive person or group to share in your process. Lying to yourself is easy. If you're accountable to other people there's more at stake and you're more likely to follow through. Admit your weaknesses so you can find strength. If you can't do it on your own then reach out to a coach, mentor, or therapist. You may need to look outside yourself or you may not. If you need more support, allow yourself to be courageous in asking for help. Be accountable to someone and be heard. Allow them to walk beside you in your venture toward wellness.

The reticular activating system (RAS) is that part of your brain determines what you notice in your life and all around you. That part of your brain helps you notice anything that relates to this goal. The brain becomes primed to get you to notice anything that relates to your goal. An example would be if someone was looking to take up mountain biking. As soon as this becomes their goal, their RAS helps them to notice any and all objects that look like a mountain bike. Now they see mountain bikes everywhere when they barely noticed them before. Your brain is primed for what you want and for your goal and you will begin to notice things around you more often that relate to getting you there if you simply create a goal. In order to remain primed, you must continue reviewing your goal daily. It's important to envision, have the reasons why you're doing it, and review the goal or goals daily.

Commit to the sixty-six days and transform your life for the better. For added motivation, make the commitment for a marathon or fitness competition at the end of the sixty-six day challenge; or commit to looking amazing at the trip you've planned out sixty-six days in advance; or make the commitment to go with your kids or your partner somewhere you've been unable to go because of your previously low energy levels.

Little things every day can make a significant impact. Don't give yourself strict rules. Look at food differently using the coping skills you've learned. Practice mindful eating at every meal. When you are about to eat, ask yourself, "What if this can nourish me?" "What if it can help my body come alive?" Practicing coping skills like mindfulness and mindful eating and engaging in behaviors that are aligned with your true identity will get you to your goal. After sixty-six days, your habits will be automatized and you will be sailing along with ease.

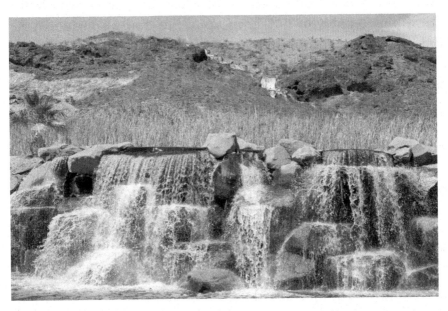

Commit to the 66 day progress. You will not arrive at the finish line because it's about making progress daily for the rest of your life. However, at the end of the sixty-six days the process will become exponentially easier because your habits and your results will be aligned with who you now believe you are and you will be habituated to the new behaviors that match with your identity. Then you can move on to asking more from yourself. You can have fun by competing with yourself. By the end of the challenge, you will feel yourself having more energy, being less tired, having better clarity with your thoughts, and experiencing improved mood. Doors will be opened that were closed before and you'll be more able to lead your ultimate life with your new habits and new body.

Chapter 11

Eating Well

We hear people say "I fast twice a week" or "I've cut out carbs." There is so much conflicting information out there. Research has shown us that dieting can do harm to your metabolism. Fasting can result in metabolic damage and it can lead to muscle tissue deterioration. Research also shows us that a life of dieting can also set people up to be more inclined to binge. Here's the bare minimum that will get you results that won't cost you so much time and indulgences:

Breakfast

Lunch

Snack

Dinner

Breakfast, lunch, snack, and dinner is a template for you for the meals you will eat during the day. It doesn't mean you cannot stray because remember...if you think "I've fallen off so I'll eat whatever I want" you are engaging in dichotomous thinking. You can easily get back on track with calorie allotment or meal planning if you let go of this all-or-nothing thinking and you commit to getting back on track. Also, it's important to remember people who are very restrictive with their diet (eating too little) set themselves up for binges (this includes people struggling with obsessive dieting and body builders getting ready for a competition). Any time you've gone four, five, or more hours without eating, stress comes along putting you in a compromising position to overeat. Going four hours without food sets you up for a ravenous state where you can easily binge so try to keep your meals to every three or three and a half hours.

Caloric deficits-counting calories- If you have a history of anorexia or bulimia and you or your treatment team believe it is too triggering for you to work out these numbers, please defer to your treatment team and allow a dietitian to crunch the numbers for you. You can have a dietitian put you on an "exchange plan" which does not involve calorie counting on your part whatsoever.

In order to lose weight you have to consume less than what your maintenance is at present. You can lose 1 to 2 lbs a week safely. I do *not* recommend consuming under 1200 calories if you are female or under 1500 calories if you are male. If you put yourself in starvation mode, then your brain has urges to binge. Your brain's main purposes is to survive. If you are in starvation mode, you will crave high caloric foods so it can store it as food. Fat is stored energy.

Breaking down the number of calories you burn each day is a scientific approach to weight loss. It is not only about weight loss, however, it's also about *optimal health*. If you are totally unaware of the magic number you may potentially be taking in too many or too few calories. Both scenarios are potentially harmful because too many calories results in excess fat stored in your body and too few calories results in starvation mode.

The key to finding a balance with food intake is knowing your active metabolic rate (AMR). Your active metabolic rate is the number of calories you burn in a day. The rates vary from one individual to the next. So, it is critical that you take the time to figure yours by breaking down the numbers.

Go here to calculate your Active Metabolic Rate: http://www.bodycalc.com/basal-metabolic-rate/bmr-amr-calculatorw to lose.

Or search "Calculate Active Metabolic Rate"

Now that you have your Active Metabolic Rate (how many calories you burn each day) you are more in control of your metabolism. If you eat more than what you burn you will gain weight. If you eat less than what you burn you will lose weight. Most experts agree that a 300 to 500 calorie deficit is safe. Remember to not go under 1200 calories if you are female or 1500 calories if you are male.

Stay ahead of the hunger. Do not skip meals. Eat according to time. Wake up within first hour ready to eat. Practice not putting yourself in a deprivation state so you can deal with frustration better. You are rewriting your history with diets, with food, with the way you think about yourself. If nothing changes then nothing changes. We need to take power back and re-establish our relationships with food. If we change what we value then we're never deprived. Indulge in quality of life.

Tricks to Slow Down and Eat Less

1. Drink a glass of water before your meal to take the edge off hunger. Allow sugar in food to hit your blood stream which triggers sense of fullness. Drink water throughout the day-with lemon. This can raise your metabolism up to three percent.
2. Avoid eating in front of TV
3. Avoid eating while standing-sitting increases your level of satisfaction from food

When a social engagement comes up you don't need to get off track completely and say "This day's a bust." The middle ground is to maintain weight calorie allotment. Go for your maintenance calorie target. You may not gain or lose but you can stay there. You may be tempted to binge and say it's a bust...in this circumstance go for the "maintain weight" mindset so even though you go over your weight loss calorie allotment you don't have to gain weight.

Change your old routines associated with food and create new routines. If you can delay craving for even three, four, or five minutes this will increase your chances of not eating during unscheduled meals or snacks. Building insight and delaying during cravings helps long-term with cravings.

Most of your meals should be aligned with your goals and some should be allotted to indulgence foods. The truth is the majority of weight loss happens as a result of improving diet. We all know that working out boosts our mood and gives us the appearance of tone.

It used to be popularly quoted by fitness experts to eat several meals throughout the day. The issue with this is that calories add up to quickly and it's not really necessary to eat numerous small meals to fuel the metabolism. Keeping your meal plan to four meals a day is a simple solution for planning your day. Remember, that if you go out and about and can't monitor every meal on a Saturday for instance, you can still maintain your goals. Try to see your weekdays as days when you are really "on it" with your meal plan. Then see your relaxation days (weekend days) as slightly off from meal plan but not actual binge episodes.

Mindful Eating

Some of us eat too fast and those of us who have a pattern of binge eating do disconnect and feel out of control during a binge. Mindless eating involves choosing food without regard to nutritional value, influence of environmental signals (TV or social situations), oversensitivity to eating triggers, not tuning into eating signals, not tuning into physical hunger signals, not tuning into taste satiety cues, and chasing flavor (if I just eat more I will get that pleasure back that was there only in the first few bites), and not being aware of fullness cues. There are techniques for becoming more mindful-more present-and centered while you are eating. In contrast to mindless eating, there is mindful eating. It is a cognitive state marked by attentional stability. One of the effects of mindful eating is that it is powerful in disengaging habitual reactions.

Mindful eating is one of the most important tools you can master to disengage from binge eating behaviors. It can actually be a lot of fun. Ready to give it a go?

Mindful Eating Script

"Eating Chocolate Mindfully"

Pick up the piece of chocolate. Look at it as if you've never seen this food before. Close your eyes and take several deep relaxing breaths. Feel the chocolate in your palm. Now place it in your other hand. Feels its weight. How does it feel between your fingers? Describe how it feels. Open your eyes. Now, lift the chocolate to your nose and smell the chocolate. What does it smell like? Place the chocolate to your lips. Feel the piece of chocolate outside of your lips. Place the chocolate inside of your mouth but don't chew yet. Notice the sensations and textures. Now begin to taste it without chewing. Experience the flavor, and the texture, and savor. Begin to chew. Notice where the chocolate is in your mouth while you're chewing it. Be aware that your body is taking in that piece of chocolate as energy. Swallow and notice any tastes or sensations that linger. Gently bring your awareness back to your breath with two or three inhales and exhales.

Use mindful eating with any and every food.

When you have an urge to binge eat, you can step back and notice the urge at a distance, watch it (urge is at an 8 on a scale of 1 to 10), and use breath to get you through. You can use this mindful eating script with any and every food. Mindful eating can become habitual if you practice over and over again. Mindful eating is a powerful tool to break binge eating patterns and become free.

Food for Mood

Food directly affects your mood. We live in a stressful life and dealing with everyday life takes its toll. The place to find mood-boosting cures can be in your kitchen. Everything we eat has the potential to change our brain chemistry and the way we feel. The brain isn't isolated from the body and it's affected by what you eat and drink just as is every other part of your body.

Certain foods contain compounds that have a powerful effect on the way that we think and feel. One of these mood foods is so powerful that it could become a tool to fight crime. In the UK, pubs were experiencing high number of bar fights. They came up with the idea of giving out chocolate at the end of the night. By 1:30 am, people begin to go home, then it's time to unveil the secret weapon. At a time of the night when fights typically break out, pubs begin to hand out chocolate. Pub-goers eat the chocolate and experience a rush of energy and a release of feel-good endorphins in the brain. Between the core hours of 1:30 am and 3 am there was a sixty-percent reduction in street violence according to the study. Foods rich in protein can make us feel alert and focused. This study is a great example of how food can directly affect the neurotransmitters in your brain which alter your mood for good and for bad.

Food for Improved Mood

Salmon & Red Grapes

Grapes have plant compounds known as polyphenols which not only promote good circulation but also help you absorb more of the good mood omega-3s in fish. Omega-3 essential fatty acids are concentrated in the brain and are needed for memory and behavior. Omega-3s also have anti-inflammatory properties that can boost your overall health. Found in seafood, walnuts, and flaxseed, Omega-3s are so powerful for lifting your mood that new studies have shown Omega-3s to be more effective than antidepressants.

Walnuts & Blueberries

Walnuts are a rich source of omega-3s that help improve cognitive functioning as well as lift mood. Blueberries contain phytochemicals known as anthocyanins that protect the brain from oxidative damage. Research has shown that together, blueberries and walnuts are even more powerful at sharpening memory and improving communication between brain cells when they are eaten together.

Tomatoes and Olive Oil

We know that tomatoes have compounds called carotenoids aka lycopene that are excellent in preventing cancer and heart disease. Tomatoes are also fat-soluble so they are more available to your body when you eat them with good fats like olive oil (which has the good mood Omega-3s in it).

Kale

Folate is the compound found in kale as well as in Swiss chard, black beans and lentils. Folate has been used for decades to treat depression. Folate intake can lead to a decrease in negative mood states and fuzzy thinking.

Chile Peppers

The capsaicin found in chile peppers has been found to protect the brain during liver failure. The hotter the pepper the more of a cancer fighter and pain reducer. While capsaicin makes our mouths burning hot, it actually cools our bodies and fights inflammation, acting like aspirin and ibuprofen. The brain has many receptors for capsaicin. Our brains respond to eating habaneros and chili peppers by releasing endorphins which can gives us a sense of calm. Capsaicin also destroys carcinogens in our food like preservatives.

Raspberries & Chocolate

When raspberries and chocolate are paired together, their disease-fighting flavonoids are even more effective at thinning the blood and improving heart health. Chocolate is also a well-known mood booster. Is it possible to eat chocolate mindfully? Definitely.

Sample Meal Plan with Good Mood Foods

Breakfast:

Chocolate and Raspberry Shake

The Recipe:

Ingredients

1 ½ Cups Water

Small Handful of Raspberries (fresh or frozen)

1 Tbl Peanut Butter

3 Teaspoons Cacao Power or Cocoa Powder

1 Banana

4-5 Small Packets of Stevia

Preparation:

Blend all ingredients in blender, pour into glass, and serve!

Lunch:

Organic Kale salad with tomatoes drizzled with 1 to 2 tbl olive oil and balsamic vinegar and side of Brazil nuts

Snack:

Walnuts and Organic Blueberries

Dinner:

Salmon, side of steamed organic spinach or kale, side of quinoa with homemade chili pepper salsa (mixed in), and side of organic red grapes

Meal Plan

Sunday

1)Breakfast:_____
2)Lunch:_____
3)Snack:_____
4)Dinner:_____

Monday

1)Breakfast:_____
2)Lunch:_____
3)Snack:_____
4)Dinner:_____

Tuesday

1)Breakfast:_____
2)Lunch:_____
3)Snack:_____
4)Dinner:_____

Wednesday

1)Breakfast:_____

2)Lunch:_____

3)Snack:_____

4)Dinner:_____

Thursday

1)Breakfast:_____

2)Lunch:_____

3)Snack:_____

4)Dinner:_____

Friday

1)Breakfast:_____

2)Lunch:_____

3)Snack:_____

4)Dinner:_____

Saturday (option for unstructured yet intuitive eating day)

1)Breakfast:_____

2)Lunch:_____

3)Snack:_____

4)Dinner:_____

See your meal plan as a template...not as a rigid schedule. If you tell yourself that you are "bad" for going off the meal plan once in a while you are only setting yourself up for more self-sabotage in the form of binge eating episodes. The purpose of a meal plan is for guidance and it is also meant to keep you full so that you're not physically deprived which can lead to impulsive eating behaviors.

How to Know When You Are Ready to *Eat Intuitively*

Dietitians are experts in the concept of intuitive eating. Intuitive eating is a basic principle that is taught in nutritional counselor classes. Babies will spit out the bottle when they are no longer hungry. However, as we age we start to lose our responses to hunger cues. You may have stopped using hunger cues by now. Intuitive eating can help body builders in post-competition that have previously been placed on a meal plan and need help eating according to hunger cues. Intuitive eating can help anyone who has a history of restrictive diets and/or overeating behaviors. Intuitive eating can help anyone who has stopped eating according to hunger cues.

Intuitive eating is the ability to listen to your body when it's hungry and eat accordingly. It's easier to get to this place (of being able to take pause when you want to eat) when you ask yourself "Am I hungry?", "Am I bored?", "Do I need comfort? or "Am I stressed?" If you already have a lot of insight and you are able to put space between you and your impulses, then it is much easier to eat intuitively.

Meal plans are one way of getting a handle on what you are eating. Counting calories or having a dietitian who will keep track of your caloric intake (if you have a history of restricting to too little calories) is another way of getting a handle on how much you eat. Additionally, using an "exchange plan" is a way that you can get a handle on what you are taking in and this method is used in most inpatient eating disorder programs. Eating intuitively is widely felt to be the most ideal method for getting a handle on eating in a balanced way.

Many people do not like to count calories or they feel triggered by counting calories. Therefore, I am going to reveal to you how to know when your hunger cues are reliable. If you feel that you will hit your calorie allotment simply by tending to your hunger cues you can try a three to four week trial. Not for just a day not for just a week you need to do it at least three to four weeks in order to prevent a full relapse.

In order to see if your hunger signals have normalized, I recommend logging/recording every time you eat intuitively as well as your calorie intake every day for at least three to four weeks. This method is the best way to know if you are able to start eating to hunger cues and begin eating intuitively. For three to four weeks, record your hunger cues then count up how many calories you've had for the day. This way you can gage how close or far off you are in your calorie allotment in order to analyze whether or not you are ready for eating intuitively. Then add up how many you've had for the week and by the end of three to four weeks assess whether or not you are hitting a comfortable range close to your ideal caloric intake. If your average is on or close to the mark, then you are ready for intuitive eating and eating according to hunger cues.

Losing weight is a very individualized process meaning what suits one person may not suit another person. If counting calories doesn't feel right for you, you may ask a dietitian for help and get on an exchange plan or you may adhere to a meal plan. If you try intuitive eating and you feel yourself slipping you may be more comfortable counting calories to stay on track. Intuitive eating is an ideal way but it's not the only way so you do not have to feel shame if you are not able to eat according to hunger cues. In fact, many people I have worked with who have conquered binge eating are still unable to simply eat when they are hungry so they stay with the plan that works for them.

Chapter 12

Working Out, Breaking Out of the Impulse to Binge, and Preventing Relapse

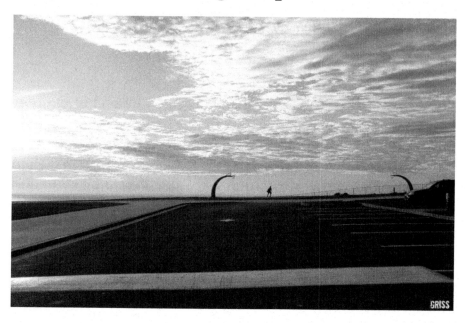

Studies show that self-esteem can be boosted and stress levels can significantly decrease by engaging in regular activity. Poor sense of self, stress, and depression directly influence a person's urge to binge eat. Research participants that have complied with regular physical activity recommendations have shown increased confidence, a stronger sense of self, and decreased stress levels.

Waking up and having a shake (as opposed to waking up and having a cigarette) is an example of a complementary behavior to exercise. Eating quinoa with avocado is a complementary behavior to exercising as opposed to eating a chili dog. So choosing and eating foods that give you fuel are complementary behaviors as they relate to being active on a particular day. Instead of skipping breakfast or eating a heavy lunch, you are choosing behaviors that are more aligned (complementary) with being physically active. This puts you in a state in which you are more likely to be active rather than inactive because your previous choices are more aligned (complementary) with working out. You are setting yourself up with your eating behaviors to be more active in your day.

The Workout Plan

I began leaning out and eventually became physical fit in order to become a certified personal trainer. I still use this workout as a standard and add variations with increases in intensity. The workout outlined for you is exactly what I was doing when I shot the cover of my first book "The Psychology Behind Fitness Motivation."

I don't like overly complex routines. Many people are so overwhelmed with complexity in their lives they don't need complexity in their workouts. This will keep it simple for you and get you results.

My workout plan is six days a week. I actually find it easier to work-out six days a week as opposed to three times or four times a week because it helps me to stay in the routine and it helps me feel like working out is a natural part of my day almost every day. Many people with a history of binge eating live in extremes (all or nothing) so making your workouts pretty much every day is a good way to feel satisfied and stay in the routine. You will find this simplified and highly effective plan for leaning out on the next page. It's called "The Secret to Shred Workout Plan."

The Secret to Shred Workout Plan

Monday: Incline walking (walking uphill or using incline treadmill) 30-45 min, 4 sets of 20 sit-ups, 3 sets of alternating lunges, 1 to 2 sets of 15 push-ups, 3 sets of bicep curls (minimum 5 lb dumbbells for women-I use 8 to 10 lb-men should use enough weight to be at failure by the end of reps), stretch

Tuesday: Incline walking 30-45 min, 4 sets of 20 sit-ups, 5 sets of 20 chair dips (works your triceps), stretch

Wednesday: Incline walking 30-45 min, 4 sets of 20 sit-ups, 3 sets of squats, 3 sets of 20 shoulder presses, hold plank position on floor for 60 seconds, stretch

Thursday: Incline walking 30-45 min, 4 sets of 20 sit-ups, 6 sets of 20 bicep curls, 1 to 2 sets of 15 push-ups, stretch

Friday: Incline walking 30-45 min, 4 sets of 20 sit-ups, 3 sets of 20

alternating lunges, 3 sets of 20 chair dips (for tricepts), stretch

Saturday: **Incline walking 30-45 min, 4 sets of 20 sit-ups, 6 sets of 15 shoulder presses, 3 sets of squats, stretch**

Sunday: **Off**

Exercise Log

This is your workout log. You can use this log to both plan out your workouts and to log what you have accomplished. Remember to have at least one day of rest.

Monday

_____
_____
_____

Tuesday

_____
_____
_____

Wednesday

_____

_____

_____

Thursday

_____

_____

_____

Friday

_____

_____

_____

Saturday

_____

_____

_____

Sunday

_____

_____

_____

If you are committing to weekend workouts *commit*. Then every Saturday and Sunday morning you are active. If you can wake up early or drive to the gym after work commit to those work week days. I still believe doing something active six days a week is the easiest way to remain in an active mode. Routine is everything. Remember it takes sixty-six days to form a new habit so allow yourself to feel out of your comfort zone just for that long. You aren't going to want to do it but you don't want to do a lot of things that you already do for others, for your work. This is the one thing that will make you happy and give you with some serious payoff. Before you know it you will be walking confidently into parties and into work. You'll be more productive, more energized, and you'll be doing more things that are aligned with who you really are as an individual.

Break Out of the Impulse to Binge

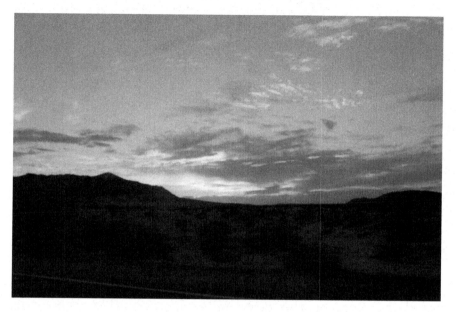

You have a pattern of sitting around on the couch and overeating or being on social media and over-snacking or coming home after a stressful day and binge eating. What I'm about to teach you will help you break that habit. This technique will help you change your destructive patterns. It's simple and it's a prescription for change.

#1 Get yourself in that destructive state that's making you depressed/anxious/frustrated...For example, you have a pattern of sitting around feeling depressed (How would you stand? What would your physiology be like?) Your head may be down, you're feeling tension in body. You are focusing on how life sucks or how things never change. Wherever you usually are in your home or at work or wherever you are when you are triggered to binge eat go there. Say the things that you say to yourself when you're in that state "I feel horrible" "I feel like a loser" "I'm not getting anywhere"... Intensely feel that emotional state. Keep affirming these negative thoughts until your physiology matches (your body is slumped, your head is down...). Whatever you usually say and feel in that state, say and feel it with intensity. Be totally immersed in this weak state.

#2 While you're feeling that emotional state, right at the peak of that feeling, do something **explosive** to jolt your nervous system. Shock your nervous system by shouting "Wake up!" Or shout a powerful statement like "I'm strong" or "Get up!" Shout it out loud and at the same time do something physical...jump up and down or spin around or pound on your chest and grunt-do something hilarious. Do anything to get up and out of the state you were in before. This is an example of pattern interruption.

#3 Now, put yourself in the state that you need to be in to feel grounded. Replace the negativity with something new and empowering. Put your shoulders back, ground yourself, center yourself, take in deep breath, smile, look up, visualize what you want, focus on your dreams, get excited about your life and how you want it to be.

You have successfully begun to interrupt the old pattern that was causing you to self-soothe with food. In order to condition yourself in a positive way you must repeat this over and over again. Whenever you find yourself in that negative state (anxious, stressed, frustrated, bored, down) which is causing you urges to binge eat, break out with your powerful pattern interruption ritual. Condition yourself by repeating it so many times that it becomes habitual. Interrupt the pattern so many times that it cannot go back. The new replacement pattern that you've created can have a dramatic impact on your life!

Relapse Prevention

Refer to what I call the 6 R's for Relapse Prevention

What is relapse prevention?

Relapse prevention is a systematic method of teaching recovering individuals to recognize relapse warning signs and to prevent returning to unwanted behaviors.

We usually hear about relapse and relapse prevention as it relates to drug and alcohol recovery. However, relapse prevention is an important concept for food addiction and binge eating recovery. Recovery is defined as abstinence plus a full return to bio/psycho/social functioning. Relapse is defined as the process of becoming dysfunctional in recovery, which leads to a return to overeating behaviors. Relapse episodes are usually preceded by a series of observable warning signs. Usually, relapse progresses from bio/psycho/social stability through a period of progressively increasing distress that leads to physical or emotional collapse. The symptoms intensify unless the individual turns to the use of alcohol or drugs or binge eating for relief.

To understand the progression of warning signs, it is important to recognize the dynamic interaction between the recovery and relapse processes. Recovery can be described as related processes that unfold in six ways:

- Abstaining from binge eating behaviors

- Separating from people, places, and things that promote binge eating, and establishing a social network that supports recovery

- Thinking rationally and engaging in positive self-talk

- Managing emotions responsibly without resorting to compulsive behavior

- Learning to change addictive thinking patterns that create painful feelings and self-defeating behaviors

- Identifying and altering the mistaken core beliefs about oneself, others, and the world that promote irrational thinking

When people who have had a stable recovery and have done well begin to relapse, they simply reverse this process. In other words, they

- Have a mistaken belief that causes irrational thoughts

- Begin to return to addictive thinking patterns that cause painful feelings

- Engage in compulsive, self-defeating behaviors as a way to avoid the feelings

- Seek out situations involving people who overeat or people who trigger them to overeat

- Find themselves in more pain or distress, thinking less rationally, and not utilizing coping skills to deal with emotions

- Find themselves in a situation in which food use seems like a logical escape from their pain, discomfort, boredom, or distress

We all have lapses (a slip rather than a full relapse) which can include overeating/binge eating behaviors. However, to avoid a full relapse in which you've gone days, weeks, or months engaging in binge eating, you can use my six R's for binge eating relapse prevention.

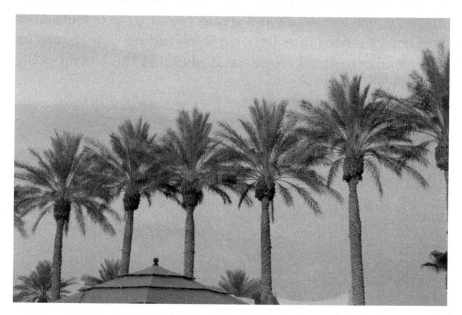

The 6 R's for Relapse Prevention:

Recognize your limits-Avoid getting into a restrictive diet-adjust your calorie allotment if it is just not enough to feel energized. Adjust your workout routine if it feels overwhelming or too intensive.

Rest-Take your rest days. We all need days off physically and mentally weekly. Prevent burnout by remembering to take at least one rest day a week with your diet and your workouts.

Reach Out-Call a supportive and positive friend or call your mentor or coach.

Refer back to Toolbox-Use all of the coping skills outlined in this book.

Routine-Quickly get back into your routine when you fall off.

Reinforcement-Reward yourself daily, weekly, and monthly. Get your hair styled by a professional, get headshots taken, get a massage, use the sauna and steam room, go to a concert, or take a trip. *Reward is as important as routine.* Put reward on your calendar to avoid relapse and maintain the body and life that you want for good.

Conclusion

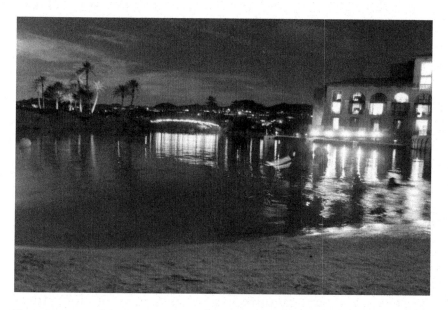

By now you've set your intention that it is a must for you to master your body and your emotions for this powerful lifestyle shift. You have the tools to engage and implement your action plan.

This process is about more than losing weight. It's about living authentically and feeling good inside so you can improve other areas of your life and gain more control. You are now conditioned to eat mindfully and to raise your standards for your physical health. Your new physical freedom will bring along with it amplified energy, strength, confidence, and a renewed interest in social engagement and activities you previously enjoyed. You were the one who had to make the decision for change and I applaud you.

A whole new level and an entirely new life is open to you now. You know what it takes for you to be free. You are in charge of your body, your mind, and your emotions. You have now turned your wants into musts. You have raised your standards. Remember that the more you turn to food the more pain you feel. Remind yourself that the more mindfully you eat the more you will engage in real life resulting in added happiness.

Enjoy the impact your lifestyle change will have on you and your family. By reinforcing these behaviors with reward and repeating them you will sustain change. The result will be an interrupted old pattern and an acquired new pattern for long-term maintenance of your lifestyle goals. I want to hear about your successes, your ups and downs, and your lasting commitment to your *musts*.

Remember that it's very hard to change a behavior when it's habitual and we don't even know what is causing the behavior. Triggers can be dealt with by utilizing the positive coping skills you have at your disposal. The result will be an interrupted old pattern and an acquired new pattern for long-term maintenance of your lifestyle goals. There's pleasure in taking control. You have new ways to alter your biochemistry, physiology, and emotional conditioning for the better. *You* have raised your standards, changed your beliefs, and adopted strategies for THE BODY YOU WANT FOR LIFE.

Congratulations!

*Photography credits for this book by Griss Noriega

Part IV

Extras

About the Author

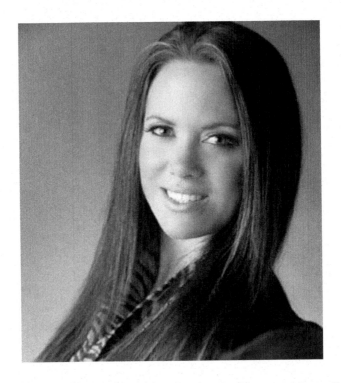

Dr. Kim Chronister specializes in health psychology with a focused expertise in Binge Eating Disorder (BED). Prior to entering the field of clinical psychology, she worked as a certified personal trainer successfully improving the lives and well-being of many clients. While pursuing her doctoral degree, she provided individual, family, couples, and group therapy to clients suffering from substance abuse, eating disorders and other issues such as anxiety and depression in residential, community, and a psychiatric facility in southern California. She has gained experience utilizing cognitive behavioral therapy (CBT) with clients struggling with eating disorders (including binge eating disorder), interpersonal issues, substance abuse, anxiety, and depressive disorders. Additionally, she uses motivational interviewing (MI) to help clients gain motivation to engage in physical activity for the benefit of decreasing stress and improving mood. Dr. Chronister uses a strength-based approach to therapy and focuses on the strengths of individuals and couples rather than pathology.

As an expert in health psychology, Dr. Kim Chronister has been asked to comment on subjects as overeating, exercise motivation, substance abuse, relationships, and numerous mental health related issues for popular magazines, books, radio shows, and documentaries. She emphasizes in her clinical practice the importance of physical fitness activity and nutrition on mood and overall well-being for individuals as well as couples.

www.DrKimChronister.com

Check out my other books

Below you'll find my books that are popular on Amazon and Kindle as well. Simply click on the link below to check them out. Alternatively, you can visit my author page on Amazon to see other my other work.

Check out the Book:

The Psychology Behind Fitness Motivation

or

Check out my Amazon author page:

Amazon Author Page: Dr. Kim Chronister

Preview of "The Psychology Behind Fitness Motivation"

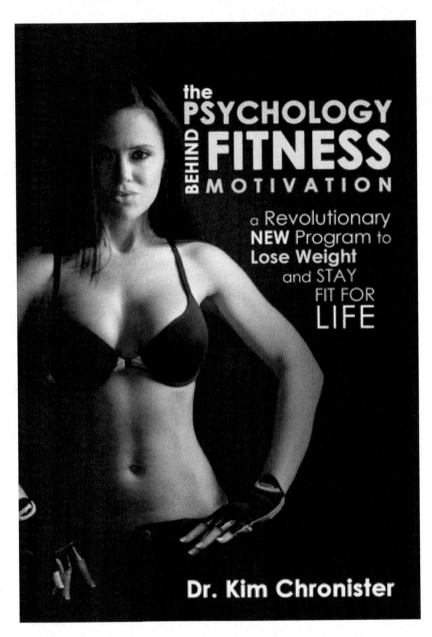

CHAPTER TWO

The Mind-Body Effects of Working-Out

Establishing the habit of exercising regularly will be one of the most important habits you will create in your life. Engaging in physical activity immediately increases levels of dopamine that helps exercise become a self-reinforcing behavior. If you continue on your fitness regimen consistently, and stay with your schedule for the most part, your brain cells in the motivation center of the brain will create new dopamine receptors. As a result, exercise will become a self-reinforcing behavior and you will gain the self-motivation that is essential in staying with a fitness regimen for life.

Depression and Exercise

Every year, Major Depressive Disorder negatively affects millions of American adults. Research for depressive issues and physical activity shows that the mental and physical gains of exercise can greatly help improve mood. Moreover, research shows that releasing feel-good neurochemicals, such as endorphins, as a product of physical fitness activity causes a feeling of wellness for body and mind. Physical fitness engagement helps greatly improve mood as well as energy and might help reduce depressive symptoms.

Despite the fact that regular physical activity may help relieve depression, only a small percentage of Americans participate in fitness activity at the recommended level As a result, many American adults don't engage in regular fitness activity and thus do not benefit from the positive mental health effects of exercise.

Although exercise can be beneficial to the mental health of clients, many
depressed individuals do not engage in enough physical activity and, therefore, are not able to benefit from the mood-elevating effects caused by regular exercise. Depressed individuals often struggle to maintain the motivation necessary to participate in regular physical activity. Although working out may be beneficial to the mental health of clients, it is difficult for most individuals to comply with a physical

activity regimen. However, making changes to one's behavior (such as engaging in physical activity) can lead to a significant improvement in mood and overall well-being.

Depression affects more millions of people globally. The lifetime risk for Major Depressive Disorder (MDD) has varied from 5 to 12 percent for adult men and 10 to 25 percent for adult women. Moreover, research suggests that people with depression are at more prone to chronic medical conditions and a higher rate of early death. Individuals with depression as well as other severe mental illnesses report worse general health and lack of exercise in their daily lives.

Currently, doctors in Britain recommend exercise first in their treatment of patients with depressive issues. However, this recommended treatment of physical activity is significantly underutilized in the United States. In addition, there's been a remarkably unfortunate increase in sedentary lifestyles from the increase in television viewing, *resulting in a large percent of adults engaging in no physical activity whatsoever*. It's no wonder why obesity is still number two when it comes to deaths that are preventable in the United States.

Many diseases, diabetes, some cancers, and depression are associated with excess weight and obesity. The individuals who experience depressive symptoms are not typically likely to participate in regular in fitness regimens. Additionally, the inverse relationship between fitness engagement and depressive symptoms has been extensively researched. Unfortunately, a lack of exercise participation has been associated with increased risk for depression.

Exercise has been shown to alleviate symptoms of depressive disorder when used as the only form of treatment. Moreover, most research shows the mood-enhancing effect of physical fitness activity is incredibly similar to traditional psychotherapy as well as psychiatric medications for depression. Combining psychiatric medications with exercise can then, in theory, have a more rapid effect on mood due to the accelerated effect of anti-depressant action (which would be beneficial considering that medications typically take several weeks to take effect). Also, exercise is a valid treatment strategy for major depressive disorder due to the fact that remaining on an exercise intervention could, in theory, be as effective as remaining on a psychiatric medications. Overall, this means that exercising along with taking antidepressants would speed up the positive mood effect and that people are likely to adhere just as much, if not more, to an exercise regimen as they would a medication regimen.

Developing a healthy lifestyle that includes physical activity is an integral part of mental well-being that is not commonly looked at in mental health treatment settings. Though upping levels of exercise can result in reducing depressive symptoms, feeling fatigued and experiencing low energy could prevent individuals with depressive disorders from remaining on fitness regimens including voluntary fitness. Empirical evidence suggests that adults, including women experiencing menopausal symptoms, can reduce their depressive symptoms and increase positive affects with physical activities such as cardiorespiratory fitness. Despite barriers such as depressed mood, fatigue, low energy, and diminished interest in activities, exercise can be beneficial to depressed individuals and may be utilized as part of a treatment program designed to enhance self-esteem and mood.

Psychological and Physiological Effects of Exercise on Mood

Several neurobiological systems may be working when clients report that physical activity helps them feel less depressed. The popular term of the
Neuro-chemical benefit of exercise is the "runner's high," that is the sense of
analgesia (pain insensitivity) as well as euphoria felt after intense exercise. Endorphins are stress hormones that relieve muscle pain and calm the brain during strenuous exercise. Moreover, endorphins produced in the brain are known to

contribute to the feeling of well-being that typically comes along with exercise. Due to the fact that plasma levels of opioids increase as a result of exercise, these opioids most likely play a role in improved mood after exercise. Thus, the endogenous opioids known as endorphins are known to be the cause of the "runner's high" phenomenon.

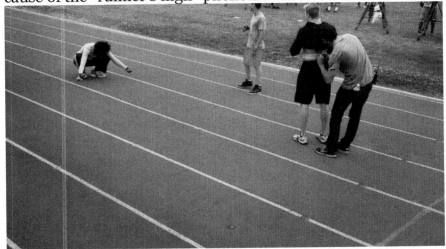

Another neurobiological system that may contribute to mood enhancement is the monoamine mechanism. Monoamines are involved in depression and many antidepressant medications increase the amounts of monoamines. Examples of monoamines include dopamine, epinephrine, serotonin, and norepinephrine. It is hypothesized that physical activity may stimulate production of monoamines. One particular monoamine, known as dopamine, plays a significant role in motivation and attention. When a person engages in physical activity, dopamine levels are increased in the brain, which results in feelings of well-being, accomplishment, and overall mood improvement. Chronic exercise increases dopamine storage in the brain and promotes the production of enzymes that form dopamine receptors in the reward center of the brain.

Physical activity regulates every one of the neurotransmitters targeted by antidepressants. Research studies showing that physical activity increases the available amount of norepinephrine as well as serotonin create interest due to the fact that most antidepressant medications, including tricyclics, SSRIs, norepinephrine and serotonin reuptake inhibitors, and MAOIs, increase norepinephrine and/or serotonin levels. Exercise immediately elevates levels of norepinephrine in the brain. In addition, serotonin is similarly affected by exercise and it plays a significant role in self-esteem, impulse control, and mood improvement. Although research suggests the factor of monoamines in major depressive disorder and great benefits of physical activity for mood, researchers have recently become aware of the problems arising out of the monoamine hypothesis with regard to depression. Among about one-third of individuals struggling with major depressive disorder, a significant portion of the already available psychiatric medications used to treat depression do not seem to be work in treating their depressive issues.

Systematic studies have been done on the most effective way of dealing with depressive symptoms that negatively affect individuals' ability to participate and benefit from physical activity. Strategies to improve physical activity participation levels that have been effective in healthy individuals can be used for those struggling with depression.

Exercise Effects on Mind and Body Simplified:

Working out affects the brain and the entire body. Since your heart is really a muscle (and responds to fitness as other muscles) it becomes larger and strengthens with regular exercise. When your heart is stronger it is more efficient. Aerobic exercise is greatly beneficial for the heart and it helps you to build endurance. In addition to getting in cardio, it is essential that you add weight training to your fitness routine. Weight training builds your muscles, which helps burn body fat, and as an added bonus it helps improve bone density. Fitness participation helps strengthen the skeletal system through bone building via osteoblast cell activation. Both resistance exercise and weight lifting can improve bone density. Exercise also helps to improve healthy levels of one's cholesterol. Blood pressure levels can also be helped through moderate forms of exercise. Moderate exercise gives an overall boost to the immune system.

When it comes to the brain, exercise helps to activate neurotransmitters
(as we discussed previously). These neurotrasmitters are "feel good"
chemicals in the brain that are released when you exercise. They include dopamine,
norepinephrine; acetylcholine, and serotonin, which helps you to calm and to sleep.
When it comes to aging, it has been shown that women who are physically active
experience less mental decline as compared to the women who refrain from engaging in regular physical activity. Therefore, regular exercise results in a better mind and a better body.

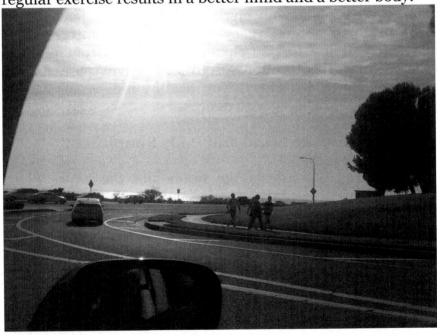

"Working-Out" Your Stress

Some of the most effective people I have met work physical activity into their routine almost every day. From speakers and authors, to actors and business owners, the successful individuals that I know choose to manage their daily stress by working out on a regular basis. They make a conscious decision and an ongoing dedication, not simply despite their busy schedules, *but because of their busy schedules.* These highly successful and effective people continue with their active lifestyles for the purpose of maintaining the energy to sustain the highest level of performance in all areas of their lives. As a result, they benefit personally, socially, sexually, and occupationally which translates into overall life satisfaction.

Situations that have the potential to cause stress (whether socially, physically, or occupationally) are an inevitable part of life. Despite the fact that you may not have the option of preventing the situation, you do hold the option to control your psychological and physiological stress levels. When stress goes untreated for long periods of time it turns into chronic stress. Chronic stress is toxic to the mind and body and has the potential to result in physical disease (such as cancer, high blood pressure, and heart problems) and mental disorders (such as anxiety disorder and depressive disorder).

Negative moods are associated with high levels of stress. A relevant mechanism for exercise-associated mood changes is called the HPA axis which is responsible for controlling your reactions to stress. The HPA axis plays a major role in depression and stress response. It regulates response in the body (caused by stress) by releasing numerous stress hormones. Additionally, the HPA axis is known to function abnormally in individuals with major depression. In response to physical (exercise) and psychological stress, stress hormones are released by the HPA axis. Although over-training increases stress hormone release, moderate training decreases the stress hormone release. Additionally, long-term participation in physical activity seems effective in minimizing a body's response to stress in the body caused by exercise as well as overall stress. Therefore, in addition to the previously discussed mechanisms for exercise-associated mood changes, the HPA axis may also play a role in mood enhancement.

Improvements in Mood and Self-Worth

Depression can result from feeling helpless and believing that there is nothing one can do to improve one's mood and/or situation. Exercise can often provide a sense of mastery and control. Low self-efficacy (the sense of being able to take control of one's life) worsens outcomes in depression. However, engagement in fitness routines has been shown to improve an individual's ability to take back control of one's life. As a result, physical activity may be an effective way for a client to feel a sense of control in his/her life. A sense of control can result in a sense of mastery, which can lead to increased self-esteem, and exercise has the potential to alleviate depression due to self-esteem enhancement. Lastly, improvement in mood may also increase the potential for a person to continue working-out due to the positive effect on self-esteem.

Recommended Guidelines for Physical Activity

A recommendation for exercise to almost every individual is unlikely to cause harm and likely to be very beneficial. In the past, what was recommended for exercise was thirty minutes of physical fitness activity (moderate intensity) for the majority of the days of the week. Currently, the weekly recommendation for physical activity (for individuals aged 18 to 65) is two and a half hours of cardio (moderate intensity) in addition to muscle strengthening (such as resistance training or weight lifting) on two or more days. Exercise and mixed exercise (aerobic and resistance) are more effective than aerobic exercise alone in reducing patient-perceived symptoms of depression.

Another notable form of exercise that has been proven to reduce symptoms of depression is "mindful" exercise. Examples of mindful exercises include Tai Chi and yoga. Studies involving adults report very significant mental and physical effects from lifestyle intervention programs that focus on mind and body exercises Tai Chi and yoga.

Walking is the number one (as far as frequency) recommended form of physical fitness activity within health care settings. Moreover, walking may be more adhered to than other exercises.

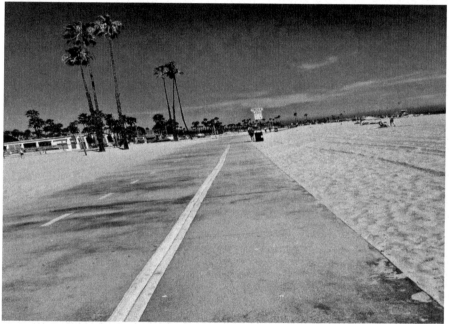

Although walking is known as the most frequent form of physical activity recommended by health care professionals, mixed exercise (aerobic and resistance) is more effective than aerobic exercise alone in reducing patient-perceived symptoms of depression. In health care settings, advice from a medical professional has the potential to lead to short-term (less than 12 weeks) increases in physical activity. However, referrals to exercise specialists can lead to long-term (up to eight months) change in both health care and community settings. It is critical for all individuals that have risk factors for cardiovascular disease to seek a medical clearance prior to participating in a fitness activity regimen.

Routine and Consistency Equals Success

No matter the form of exercise you choose (the one recommended to you in this book, or a physical hobby, or a combination thereof) the key to making your motivation last and maintaining your ideal body is CONSISTENCY! Set the amount of days you will be active and stick to your routine. The fitness regimen that will fit into your schedule is the one you will embrace and be able to continue in the long-term.

Research shows that approximately half of those who begin a new fitness regimen drop out within six months to a year. *One of the major reasons why people fail to keep up with their fitness regimens is that they begin a workout that is not appropriate for their fitness level.* As a result, they feel that they are not good enough to stick with the work out and they quit. You may have experienced an intense workout that made you vomit afterwards (literally) and left you feeling defeated. Remember, when you begin my workout regimen (later in the book) that it is more important to do some of the workout consistently than nothing or sometimes. I have had many clients who (despite not being in the mood and having busy schedules) made sure they did at least part of their workout when it was scheduled.

Establishing the habit of exercising regularly (even if it is some of the workout and you remain on schedule) will be among the most essential habits you will create for yourself. Since engaging in exercise immediately increases levels of dopamine, exercise will become a self-reinforcing behavior for you. When you continue on your fitness regimen on a consistent basis, and stay with your schedule for the most part, your brain cells in the motivation center of the brain will create new dopamine receptors. As a result, you will gain the self-motivation that is essential in staying with a fitness routine for life.

You can use the techniques in this program to have fitness motivation for life. You will also accomplish something more powerful: you will prove to yourself that you have the power to change your thoughts and behaviors and improve your mood. This power will increase your confidence and you will view yourself in a new and incredible way. You will also empower yourself with the tools that will help you achieve greater control of your mind, body, and quality of life.

[Click here to check out the rest of (The Psychology Behind Fitness Motivation) on Amazon](#)

Or Search "Fitness Motivation" on Amazon